HIGH BLOOD PRESSURE

FOOD · FACTS · RECIPES

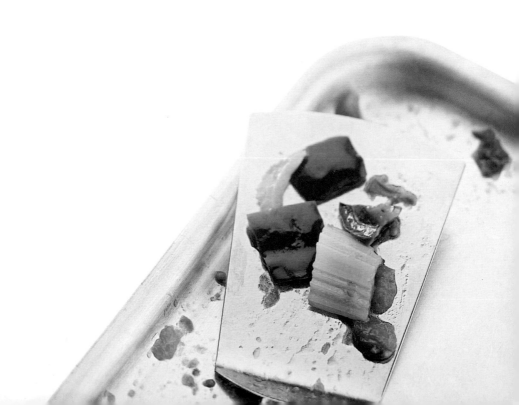

hamlyn

HIGH BLOOD PRESSURE

FOOD • FACTS • RECIPES

ANGIE JEFFERSON AND FIONA HUNTER

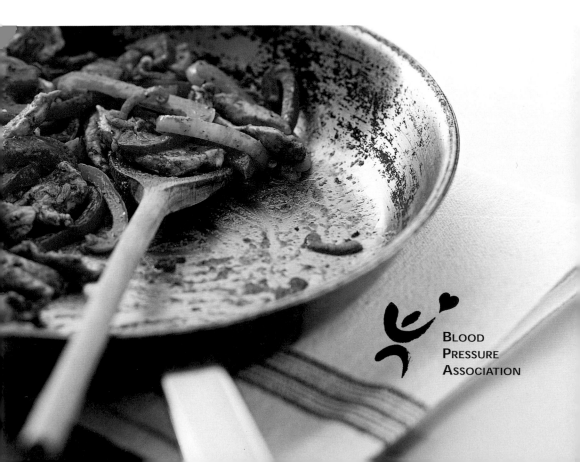

BLOOD
PRESSURE
ASSOCIATION

The Blood Pressure Association (BPA) is a U.K. organization for people affected by high blood pressure. High blood pressure is a risk factor for stroke, heart disease, kidney failure, and some types of dementia, which means that if you have high
blood pressure you are more likely to have one of these conditions than some one who's blood pressure is not raised. The BPA provides information and support to help people to manage and lower their blood pressure, as well as raising awareness among the general population of the importance of high blood pressure.

High blood pressure rarely has any symptoms and the only way to find out if you have it is to have your blood pressure measured.

The BPA ensures that people with high blood pressure, as well as health professionals, help them to develop and write all of their information so that they can help you to successfully manage your condition.

Blood Pressure Association
60 Cranmer Terrace
London
SW17 0QS
U.K.
Website: www.bpassoc.org.uk

CAUTIONS

Nutritional analysis is provided for each recipe and given per serving. Where a recipe has split servings (e.g. "serves 6–8"), the analysis is given for the first figure.

People with known nut allergies should avoid recipes containing nuts or nut derivatives and vulnerable people should avoid dishes containing raw or lightly cooked eggs.

This book is not intended to replace medical care under the direct supervision of a qualified doctor. Before embarking on any changes in your health regime, consult your doctor. While the advice and information are believed to be accurate and true at the time of going to press, neither the author nor the publisher can accept legal responsibility or liability for any errors or omissions that may have been made.

Ovens should be preheated to the specific temperature. If using a fan-assisted oven, follow the manufacturer's instructions for adjusting the time and temperature. Grills should also be preheated.

Both metric and imperial measurements are given for the recipes. Use one set of measurements only, not a mixture of both.

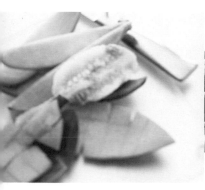
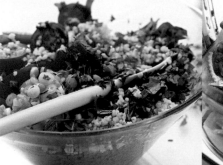

An Hachette UK Company
www.hachette.co.uk

First published in Great Britain in 2005 by
Hamlyn, a division of Octopus Publishing Group Ltd
Endeavour House, 189 Shaftesbury Avenue,
London, WC2H 8JY
www.octopusbooks.co.uk
www.octopusbooksusa.com

This edition published in 2013

Copyright © Octopus Publishing Group Ltd 2005

Distributed in the US by Hachette Book Group USA
237 Park Avenue, New York NY 10017 USA

Distributed in Canada by Canadian Manda Group, 165
Dufferin Street, Toronto, Ontario, Canada M6K 3H6

ISBN: 978-0-600-62626-8

Printed and bound in China

10 9 8 7 6 5 4 3 2 1

contents

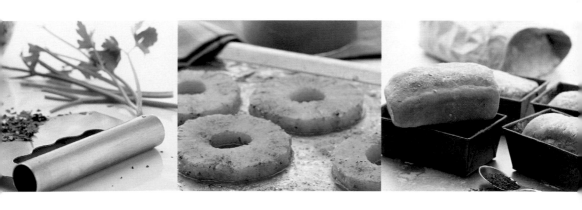

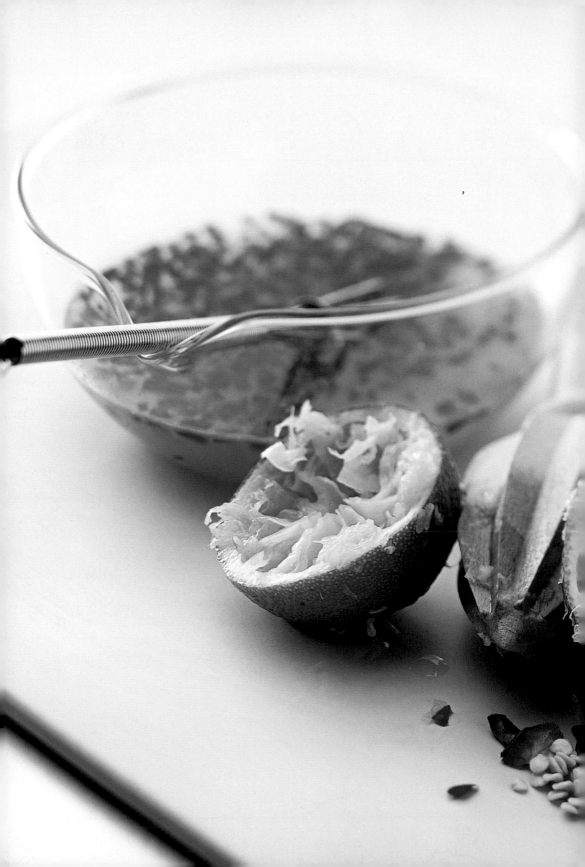

introduction

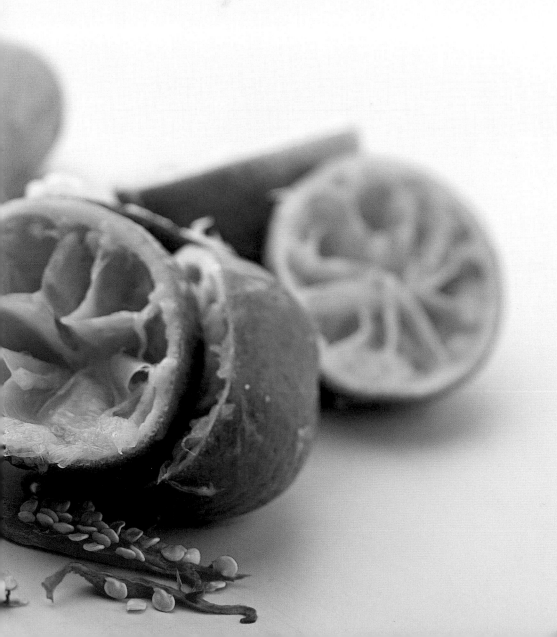

introduction

This book has been written for the many people who already have high blood pressure, as well as for those whose genetics or lifestyle make them potential candidates for this condition. High blood pressure, also known as hypertension, is common, affecting one in three women and two in five men in the U.S.A., the U.K., and in Australia. However, many people are unaware that they have it. If you have been diagnosed with high blood pressure, you have the advantage of knowing your blood pressure measurement and being able to do something to look after your health.

"According to the World Health Organization, high blood pressure is a key factor in about half the cases of heart disease worldwide"

The impact of high blood pressure

The main reason for concern is that high blood pressure is a major risk factor for stroke, heart attack, and heart failure. The *Journal of Human Hypertension* (2003) and American Heart Organization statistics (2001) estimate that 47,000 people in the U.S.A. and 62,000 people in the U.K. die unnecessarily each year because of poor blood pressure control.

Look after yourself

Tackling each of the different aspects of your diet and lifestyle addressed on the following pages should help you lower your blood pressure—and the more of them that you try, the greater the overall effect is likely to be. For some people this may mean that they don't need medication to control their blood pressure. Others may still need medication, but possibly at a lower dose than would otherwise be necessary. Either way, use the knowledge gained from this book to keep yourself in tip-top health and your blood pressure under control. Even if you don't currently have high blood pressure, following the advice given here should help you avoid the rise in blood pressure that tends to happen as we get older.

Blood pressure: the facts

Blood pressure is the force of the blood against the walls of the blood vessels. Without blood pressure blood vessels would collapse, blood would stop flowing, and the body would not receive the oxygen and nutrients vital to life. Blood pressure varies naturally, rising and falling at different times of the day and in response to mental and physical exertions. In general, blood pressure tends to be highest in the mornings and lowest at night.

What is high blood pressure?

High blood pressure occurs when, as the name suggests, the blood pressure rises and then stays high. This is dangerous to health because the heart has to work harder, and the risk of developing a heart attack, stroke, or vascular dementia—impaired blood supply to the brain causing progressive loss of brain function—increases. High blood pressure damages the blood vessels, making them less flexible and narrowing them, leading to damage to the kidneys, eyes, heart, and brain. The damage to the blood vessels can also lead to clots, increasing the risk of heart attack and stroke, and sometimes to the blood vessels bursting, also causing strokes. It is therefore important that everyone has their blood pressure

WHY CONTROL YOUR BLOOD PRESSURE?

Untreated high blood pressure can lead to:

- Increased risk of stroke or heart attack
- Damage to the heart, brain, or eyes
- Heart failure
- Angina
- Kidney disease
- Vascular dementia

"If you have high blood pressure, reducing it by just 5mmHg can reduce your risk of suffering a heart attack by about 20 percent"

checked at least every couple of years, and more frequently if it has ever been high or there is a family history of high blood pressure.

Most of the time there are no symptoms of high blood pressure and it is diagnosed only during a routine checkup. A very small number of people may suffer from headaches or nose bleeds, but the only sure way of knowing whether your blood pressure is high is to have it measured.

The causes of high blood pressure

Often there is no single cause of high blood pressure, it just happens. However, a range of things contribute to high blood pressure. These include having an unhealthy diet that contains too much salt and salty foods, drinking too much alcohol, and being overweight or obese.

Genetics also plays a part. If either or both of your parents had high blood pressure you are more likely to get it as well. Also, if you are of African descent you are more likely to suffer high blood pressure than Caucasians.

Some people may have high blood pressure caused by health problems such as kidney disease and diabetes, or caused by certain medications prescribed to treat ulcers, arthritis, or depression.

What should my blood pressure be?

Blood pressure is measured in millimeters of mercury and expressed as mmHg. The ideal blood pressure is considered to be below 120/80mmHg. The top figure of the fraction (called systolic pressure) is when the heart beats, contracting and squeezing blood around the body, and the bottom figure of the fraction (called diastolic pressure) is when the heart is relaxed, between heartbeats. High blood pressure is diagnosed when these levels consistently rise above 140/90mmHg. It is possible for one level to be high and the other to be within normal limits—this is still regarded as high blood pressure. The levels for high blood pressure are the same whether you are male or female, young or old.

Treating high blood pressure does not necessarily mean taking medication. For many people making changes to their lifestyle or body weight may be enough to bring blood pressure down to normal levels.

Low blood pressure

Although high blood pressure is far more common, there are some individuals who have low blood pressure. Like high blood pressure, low blood pressure tends to have no symptoms. However, it can cause dizziness or even fainting after getting up quickly from sitting or lying down, especially in older people. There is usually no need to treat low blood pressure.

Putting it all together

Many studies have examined the effect on blood pressure of changing a single lifestyle or dietary factor. However, one study carried out in the U.S.A. (Appel *et al*, 2003) has clearly shown that the most effective approach to blood pressure management is to combine several factors—weight control, reduced salt intake, eating more fruit and vegetables, increased physical activity, and a limited alcohol intake. Almost 70 percent of the study's participants reduced their blood pressure from high to normal by taking this combined approach over a six-month period.

Simple ways to lower your blood pressure…

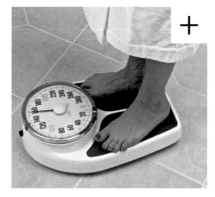 +

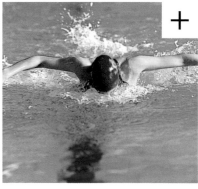 +

+ Reduce your salt intake
+ Eat at least "five-a-day"
+ Limit the alcohol you drink
+ Control your weight
+ Increase your physical activity

salt and blood pressure

Salt is an important factor affecting blood pressure. A high intake of salt is likely to push blood pressure up. From studies of populations rather than individuals, it is known that those populations whose diets contain large amounts of salt (such as the typical diet in the U.S.A., the U.K., Europe, and Australia) tend to have higher average blood pressures than those whose diets are low in salt. Where salt intakes are high, blood pressure typically increases with age, an effect not seen among low-salt eating populations.

THE DANGERS OF SALT

A diet high in salt can:

- Raise blood pressure
- Cause water retention
- Worsen osteoporosis
- Be implicated in stomach cancer
- Affect asthma
- Increase the risk of kidney disease

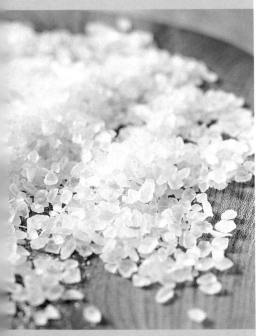

Salt sensitivity

It is thought that some people may be more sensitive to salt in their diet. At present scientists cannot distinguish the more "salt-sensitive" individuals from those who are not, but some studies have found a higher frequency of salt sensitivity in people with high blood pressure, people who are obese, have diabetes, kidney problems, or are of African descent. The more salt-sensitive individuals will find that reducing their salt intake will have great and rapid effects on their blood pressure, while for those who are less salt sensitive, cutting their salt intake will have smaller, slower effects. What *is* clear is that the majority of us consume far higher amounts of salt than we actually need to eat and this is likely to be raising blood pressure to some extent in all of us. The expert consensus therefore is that we should all be taking steps to reduce our daily salt intake—from checking labels on processed foods to reducing what we add to cooking.

Salt or sodium

Some manufacturers label food with sodium content rather than salt. It is easy to work out the conversion: 0.25 g (250 mg) is the amount of sodium contained in 1 g of salt. Sodium, the harmful constituent of salt, is also found in such ingredients as baking powder and soy sauce.

The DASH evidence

One of the most informative studies on the effects of salt on blood pressure is the DASH (Dietary Approaches to Stop Hypertension) trial, which was published in the U.S.A. in 2001. The trial showed that changing to a diet rich in fruit and vegetables, low-fat dairy foods, and foods reduced in saturated and total fat significantly reduced blood pressure.

The DASH-Sodium trial compared the effects of low, medium, and high salt intake on blood pressure while eating either a typical American high-fat diet, or the healthier DASH diet. The low-salt diet contained 3.7 g salt, the medium-salt diet 6 g salt, and the high-salt diet 8.2 g salt per day (which is the low end of current typical salt intakes in the U.S.A. and U.K.). Reducing salt intake lowered blood pressure in both the American and the DASH diet groups, and the lower the salt intake the lower the blood pressure became.

The great news was that the people with the highest starting blood pressures had the greatest falls with salt reduction, no matter whether they were following the typical American or DASH diet plan. Changing from a typical Western, high-fat diet to one rich in fruit, vegetables, and cereal foods, with no change to salt intake, resulted in a fall in blood pressure. The study showed that reductions in blood pressure were greatest at each level of salt intake for those eating the healthier DASH diet, showing that combining a reduced-salt intake with healthier eating had the greatest impact on lowering blood pressure.

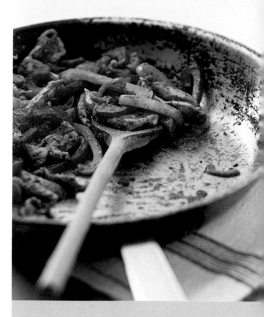

"Salt intake is considered to have a direct adverse effect on blood pressure—generally, the more salt you eat the higher your blood pressure will be. Cutting down on salt in cooking and at the table, and eating less salty foods is therefore an important step toward better health"

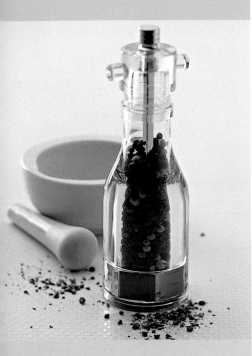

REEDUCATE YOUR TASTEBUDS

Instead of using salt at home:

- Place a pepper mill on the table instead of the salt shaker

- Use plenty of fresh or dried herbs – try adding a sprig of fresh mint to the pan of potatoes during cooking, stirring fresh chopped parsley or chives or small amounts of wholegrain mustard into mashed potato or using grated ginger to flavor soups or casseroles

- Be more adventurous with spices, chili, and garlic

- Marinate meats and fish in lemon or lime juice before cooking

How much salt should we eat?

Current typical salt intakes throughout the Western world are far higher than is considered healthy—the Intersalt study (studying 10,000 people in 32 countries) has shown that average intakes of salt are typically around 8–10 g per day. Both adults and children are generally consuming two to three times the amount of salt advised. The World Health Organization recommends a salt intake of no more than 5 g (equal to 1.2 g of sodium) per day, while recommendations in the U.S.A. and U.K. are for no more than 6 g per day (about 1 teaspoon, 1.5 g sodium).

Reducing the risks to health

Some experts have predicted that reducing current salt intakes by 3 g per day would result in a 13 percent reduction in strokes and a 10 percent reduction in heart disease. A more extreme reduction of 9 g per day has been predicted to potentially reduce strokes by one third and heart disease by one quarter. If these figures are applied to the U.K. population this is equivalent to preventing around 20,500 stroke deaths and 31,400 heart-disease deaths each year. Most of us would find it difficult to keep our salt intakes this low; however any reduction in salt intake could significantly reduce risks to our health.

Change your habits

For most of us, around three quarters of the salt that we eat comes from processed food, and the remaining quarter from the salt we add at home when cooking and at the table. Two thirds of us regularly add salt to our cooking and more than half of us often add salt to our food at the table. So we can immediately cut salt by a quarter (1.7 g per day) by not using salt at home.

In the long term the healthiest option is simply to give up adding salt. If at the moment you always add salt to your food, your tastebuds will be adapted to a salty taste. If you stop adding salt, food may taste a little different at first but you will adapt to these new flavors within two or three weeks. You may find it easier to simply cut out salt and wait for your tastebuds to adapt or, if you find this too hard, an alternative would be to cut down gradually over a few weeks until you give up salt completely. Enjoying salt is purely a matter of habit—and all habits can be changed if you persevere.

If you cannot do without salt at all it is probably more effective to put a tiny amount in the cooking for flavor and keep the salt shaker off the table, rather than skipping the salt in cooking and then sprinkling salt onto your food later. By doing it this way you should be able to use less salt. Rock salt, sea salt, celery and garlic salt are still salt and so the same advice applies to these.

Sources of salt in the diet

Cereal foods such as bread and breakfast cereals are one of the biggest sources of salt in the diets of both adults and children, but this does not mean that intake of these should be reduced or avoided. These foods are a staple part of the diet and valuable sources of carbohydrates, dietary fiber, and a wide range of vitamins and minerals. Many manufacturers are taking steps to reduce the amount of salt being added to these foods, which will help to reduce salt intakes over the next few years. Comparing labels between products will allow you to choose the brands containing the lowest amounts of sodium.

Meat and meat products are the second biggest source of salt in the diet, with processed meats such as burgers, sausages, and pies providing as much salt as cured meats like bacon or ham. Choosing fresh meats rather than processed, breaded, or preshaped could reduce salt intakes by around 1 g per day.

COMMERCIAL ALTERNATIVES TO SALT

Mineral salts, which contain a mixture of potassium and sodium, are widely available. These are an alternative if you really can't do without salt on your food, but still try to limit the amount that you use. Mineral salts should not be used by young children, anyone with kidney problems, or the frail elderly, as the high potassium content could have harmful effects.

LOW-SALT ALTERNATIVES

It is worth taking time to compare the salt or sodium content in foods: health food stores, and some supermarkets, are beginning to provide low-salt or no-salt alternatives to such foods as bread, cereals, and canned vegetables.

10 easy ways to reduce your salt intake…

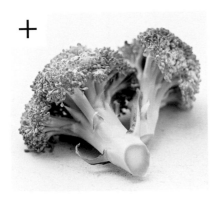

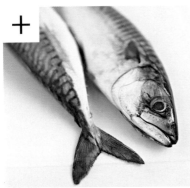

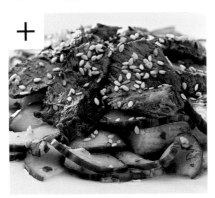

1 Choose "low-salt," "no-added salt," or "salt-free" processed foods by checking that they contain a maximum 0.25 g (250 mg) sodium or 1 g salt per 100 g.

2 Buy plain fresh or frozen vegetables or choose those canned with "no added salt."

3 Use fresh chicken, fish, and lean meats rather than canned, smoked, or processed types.

4 Limit smoked and cured foods, such as ham, bacon, and smoked kippers.

5 Choose canned fish, such as tuna or salmon, in water or sunflower oil rather than in brine.

6 Cut back on ready meals as these can often be high in salt.

7 Stock cubes and gravy granules are high in salt, so choose low-sodium varieties or cut down on how often you use them.

8 Limit relishes and sauces—use homemade salsa or guacamole as healthier options.

9 Ready-made soups can be high in salt so try making your own instead.

10 Take-out foods can be high in sodium, especially Chinese food where monosodium glutamate and soy sauce may also have been used. If you regularly order a take-out from a local outlet, try asking the staff whether they usually add salt and whether less can be used for your order.

Check the salt content

Salt is made up of sodium and chloride, and it is the sodium that affects blood pressure. Some food labels give the amount of sodium in a food—a useful comparison is to know that seawater, which tastes unpleasantly salty, contains 1 g sodium per 100 g.

Salt savings

With a few careful choices it is easy to lower your salt intake. Remember lots of small savings all add up, so save on salt wherever you can. The aim for all of us is to reduce salt intake by at least 3 g per day.

REPLACE	WITH	SALT SAVED
2 ounces dry roast peanuts	2 ounces unsalted cashew nuts	3.9 g
2 slices of ham	2 slices of fresh roast turkey	2 g
1 teaspoon salt in cooking	$^1/_2$ teaspoon salt	2.5 g
Take-out stir-fry vegetables	Home-cooked stir-fry vegetables	0.7 g
Serving of canned corn or peas in salted water	Serving of frozen corn or peas	0.7 g
Small can of ordinary baked beans	Small can of reduced-sugar, reduced-salt baked beans	1.1 g
Take-out French fries (medium portion)	Oven fries	0.7 g
Serving of smoked salmon	Broiled salmon steak	4.6 g
Breaded cod steak	Broiled plain cod steak	1.0 g
2 broiled pork sausages	1 broiled pork loin chop	2.5 g
Frozen beef grillsteak, cooked	Ground beef, dry-fried	1.6 g
2 bacon slices	2 reduced-salt bacon slices	1.4 g
4 Graham crackers	4 rye crispbreads	1.0 g
$3^1/_2$ ounces cheddar cheese	$3^1/_2$ ounces fresh mozzarella	0.8 g
Processed cheese spread	Low-fat cream cheese	0.5 g
Cheddar cheese and relish sandwich	Chicken salad sandwich	2.7 g
1 tablespoon ordinary margarine spread	1 tablespoon low-salt margarine spread	0.3 g

potassium

The mineral potassium plays a role in ensuring our good health, helping to maintain strong bones, allowing normal nerve function, and controlling blood pressure. It also helps to counteract the effects of salt on blood pressure.

"The balance between the amount of sodium and potassium in the diet has a direct relationship to blood pressure levels"

Potassium is a mineral that has many functions in the body, such as helping to control blood pressure and reduce the risk of developing heart disease and strokes, and the transmission of all nerve impulses.

One important effect of potassium is its role in helping to reduce sensitivity to salt in the diet and prevent rises in blood pressure as a result of salt intake. The balance between the amount of sodium and potassium in the diet has a direct relationship to blood pressure levels. Studies carried out in the U.S.A. have shown that among men given a diet low in potassium, salt sensitivity was relatively common— affecting almost four fifths of African-Americans and

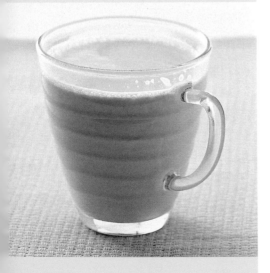

one quarter of Caucasians. However, when potassium intake was increased to that of a more typical American diet the numbers of salt-sensitive individuals fell to half among African-Americans and one fifth of the Caucasians. A much higher potassium intake was needed to reduce salt sensitivity among the African-Americans in the study.

Numerous other studies have also found a direct relationship between potassium intake (which primarily comes from eating fruit and vegetables) and blood pressure levels. It is better to obtain nutrients from the correct foods than to take supplements.

Current recommendations

Current recommendations in the U.S.A. have suggested that potassium intakes should be 4.7 g per day. Less recently published recommendations in the U.K. are to increase intake of potassium from 3 g per day to 3.5 g per day. U.K. dietary data show that potassium intakes remain around the lower level of 3 g per day and that steps still need to be taken to correct this dietary deficiency.

Potassium-rich foods:

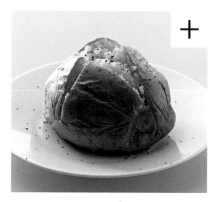

+

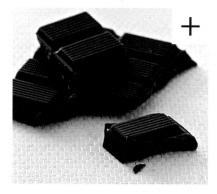

+

+ All fruit: especially bananas, melons, apricots, rhubarb, kiwi fruit, pears, black currants, citrus fruit, dried fruit, and fruit juices
+ Vegetables: especially potatoes (particularly those baked in their skins), mushrooms, squash and pumpkin, beets, pulses (including low-salt baked beans), and tomato juice
+ Dark chocolate and cocoa (in moderation)
+ Malted milk drinks

"five-a-day"

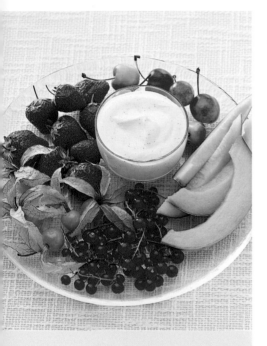

Eating "five-a-day"—at least five portions of a variety of fruit and vegetables a day—can help to significantly reduce the risk of heart disease, stroke, and some cancers, making this one of the easiest, but most effective steps to take to improve our health. Fruit and vegetables are rich sources of fiber, vitamins, and minerals, including potassium, which helps to reduce blood pressure, as well as a whole range of antioxidants vital to maintaining great health.

"More than 'five-a-day' helps keep high blood pressure at bay"

More than five

You might think you eat plenty of fruit and vegetables, but the latest surveys show that less than one in seven people achieve the goal of eating "five-a-day." On average we are managing to eat just three portions each day. And younger people are the worst, with four out of five of those aged 16–24 years eating fewer than three portions of fruit and vegetables a day.

In terms of blood-pressure control, the usual recommendation is not just to eat "five-a-day" but to eat between seven and nine portions of fruit and vegetables each day. So in simple terms, however many fruit and vegetables you are eating the chances are that you probably need to eat more.

According to the British Hypertension Society, increasing your consumption of fruit and vegetables from two to seven portions each day has been shown to lower blood pressure by 7/3mmHg. When this is combined with other dietary measures such as eating more low-fat dairy foods, falls in blood pressure are larger, averaging 11/6mmHg.

Variety

To get the maximum benefits, our bodies need a variety of different types of fruit and vegetables as they all contain different combinations of nutrients. Think about the different colors of fruit and vegetables. Each color contains different antioxidants and nutrients, so a basic guide is to try to eat a rainbow of fruit and vegetables over a week.

The fruit and vegetables contained in convenience foods (and take-out meals), such as ready meals, pasta sauces, soups, and desserts, can all count toward your "five-a-day." However, convenience foods can also be high in added salt, sugar, and fat, so always check the nutrition information on food labels.

What counts as a portion?

One portion of fruit or vegetables is equivalent to 3 ounces, not counting the pith, seeds, skin, or any other part that you do not eat—see the examples in the box, right. These portion sizes are for adults. Children should also eat at least five portions of fruit and vegetables each day, but the portion sizes may be smaller for them.

Dried fruit counts toward "five-a-day," as does 100 percent fruit or vegetable juice, but you can only count juice as one portion each day, no matter how much you drink. This is because juicing removes much of the fiber, affects the vitamin content, and "squashes" the natural sugars out of the cells that normally contain them.

Similarly, beans and other pulses such as lentils and chickpeas (garbanzo beans) can only count once a day, however much you eat. Beans and pulses contain fiber, but they don't provide the same mixture of vitamins, minerals, and other nutrients as fruit and vegetables. Potatoes are generally considered a "starchy" food (like rice, pasta, and bread), and so don't count toward "five-a-day."

Simple ways to get "five-a-day"…

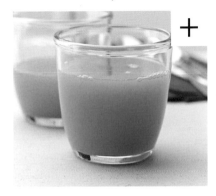

+

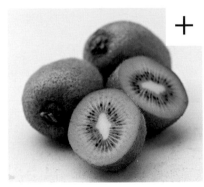

+

+ ½ large grapefruit or mango
+ 1 slice of melon or pineapple
+ 2 satsumas, plums, or kiwi fruit
+ 1 banana, pear, peach, or apple
+ a handful of grapes or berries
+ 1 tablespoon dried fruit
+ 3½ ounce-glass of 100 percent fruit or vegetable juice
+ 3 tablespoons cooked carrots, peas, or corn
+ 1 dessert bowl of mixed salad or vegetable soup

12 easy ways to eat more fruit and vegetables…

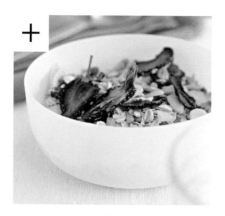

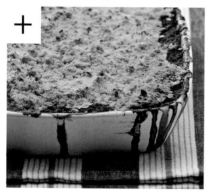

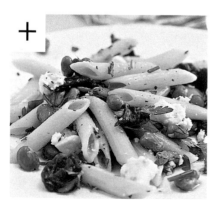

1 Slice fresh fruit or sprinkle dried fruit over a bowl of breakfast cereal.

2 Drink a glass of pure juice or a fruit smoothie every day.

3 Pep up sandwich fillings with extra salad or fruit, for example lean meat with salad or grapes, and peanut butter with banana.

4 Instead of chips serve vegetable crudités with a tomato salsa or minted yogurt and cucumber dip.

5 Serve an extra type of vegetable with your main meal.

6 Cook carrots or rutabaga with potatoes and mash them together.

7 Add frozen vegetables to rice or pasta during cooking.

8 Try new salad combinations, for example coleslaw with raisins and walnuts; apple, walnut, and celery; or corn and bell peppers.

9 Add extra vegetables to convenience meals—pile pizza with extra bell peppers, mushrooms, and tomatoes or cook some frozen vegetables at the same time as a microwave dinner.

10 Stuff a cored apple or pitted peach with dried fruit, then bake and serve with custard or yogurt.

11 Fill pancakes with stewed or canned fruit, or make a fruit crumble using lots of fruit and a thin layer of topping.

12 Top a meringue base with lots of summer fruits and just a small amount of cream.

alcohol and blood pressure

Drinking alcohol is something that many of us enjoy, and in moderation it poses no risk to health. However, it is very easy to slip into the habit of drinking too much, especially as most wines and beers today have a higher alcohol content than in the past, and serving measures have also increased in size.

Sensible drinking

A number of studies have shown the effect of alcohol consumption on blood pressure, with non-drinkers generally having slightly lower blood pressures than people who drink more than a small amount. Blood pressure rises both with acute large intakes (for example binge drinking on a Friday or Saturday evening) and with a habitually high intake of 4 or more units of alcohol per day. Both acute drinking and habitually drinking too much can increase the risk of suffering a stroke. On the other hand, moderate intakes of 1–2 units of alcohol each day may help to protect against heart disease by increasing HDL (good) cholesterol levels.

With high blood pressure you can still drink within sensible limits—which means no more than 2–3 units for a woman or 3–4 units for a man on any single day. Many wines and beers now state how many units are in each bottle or can, so you can easily check your intake of alcohol units.

"If you have high blood pressure and you drink, it is fine to carry on, as long as you drink in moderation and avoid binge drinking"

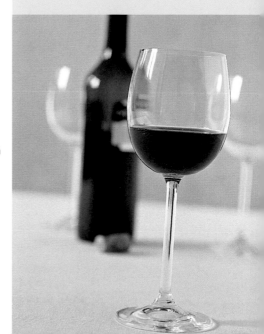

weight control

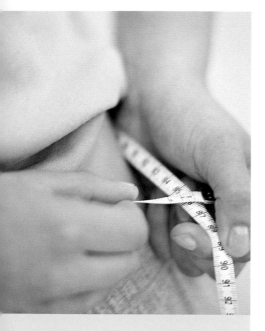

Being overweight is a major factor contributing to high blood pressure, placing a strain not only on the heart, but on all other parts of the body as well. Losing excess weight is one of the most effective ways to get your blood pressure to fall. Every 2¼ pounds of weight lost can, on average, result in a fall of 2.5mmHg systolic and 1.5mmHg diastolic blood pressure. For some people losing weight may be all that is necessary to get their blood pressure back to normal levels.

Where you carry your excess weight also makes a difference. Studies have shown that an apple shape (where the waist is bigger than the hips) is more damaging to health than a pear shape (where the hips are bigger than the waist). This is because the fat carried around the abdomen has an affect on a range of risk factors for heart disease, including raising blood pressure and blood sugar levels.

"The numbers of overweight people have increased dramatically throughout the world over the past 20 years, such that six in ten adults in the U.S.A., five in ten adults in the U.K., and four in ten adults in France, Italy, Denmark, and Australia are now overweight or obese"

Slowly does it

Losing weight slowly and steadily—1–2 pounds per week—is the most successful way to do it and an effective way to lower blood pressure. Losing weight slowly means that you are more likely to be breaking down body fat and not straining the metabolism by forcing the body to break down lean tissues, such as muscle, as well. In addition, the benefit of losing weight slowly means that you are more likely to keep it off.

The technical bit

Successful weight loss comes from understanding how your body works and the energy that you are taking in—in other words the "food versus energy" balance. Each pound of body fat contains 3500 calories, so in order to lose 1 pound in a week you will need either to eat 500 fewer calories each day or to burn off 500 calories more. A bit of both usually works best. It is simply a case of knowing what you are trying to achieve and then doing the arithmetic.

While that sticky cake or chocolate bar may look tempting it will satisfy your tastebuds for only a few moments, and will not truly satisfy your hunger. There are no good or bad foods in a healthy diet, but some are more calorie-dense than others so it makes sense to keep these as treats. Plan to eat sensible meals with lots of fruit and vegetables, and then plan in some extra treats to look forward to as well. Work out just when a treat will mean most to you, and what that treat will be—and then enjoy it to the full!

Recognize the difficult times

While there are no rules in weight loss about eating after 6 p.m., this is a time to be aware of, as we often eat our largest meal of the day during the evening and it is also the most common time for snacking as well. These combined facts make it easy to consume a large part of our daily calories in just a few hours of the day. Alcohol intake is another key factor here as well, as it is easy to fall into the habit of drinking every evening. While not necessarily harmful in itself, drinking most days will quickly add calories and slow down weight loss.

DO I NEED TO LOSE WEIGHT?

Don't worry about the scales, measuring your waist will quickly tell you whether you have a few pounds to lose. For men a waist measurement greater than 37 inches and for women a waist measurement greater than 32 inches requires weight loss.

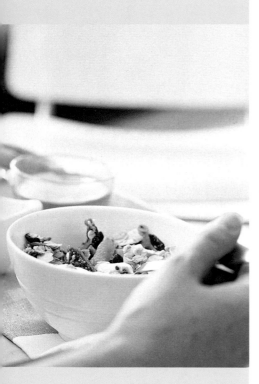

10 steps to successful weight loss

1 Always eat breakfast to wake up the body and brain, and boost your metabolism in the morning.

2 Eat at least five servings of different fruit and vegetables every day—they are great for your blood pressure, are packed with nutritional goodies, and are filling as well.

3 Choose a lower-fat spread for your toast and spread it thin.

4 Avoid snacking out of pure habit. If you truly are hungry go ahead and eat—but try some fruit instead of a chocolate bar. If you are eating because you are bored, fed up, or lonely do something else instead such as read a book, take a bath, or go for a walk.

5 Limit your intake of calorie-containing drinks— the body does not easily recognize energy in liquid form, allowing extra calories to be taken in. Cut down on sugar in hot drinks—choose water or low-calorie soft drinks, or try fruit or herbal teas instead.

6 Avoid alcohol. It is full of calories and can actually stimulate your hunger, meaning that you eat more as well.

7 Cut down on fat whenever you can, especially saturated fat (animal fats and certain vegetable oils). Cut visible fat off meat, buy lower-fat dairy foods, avoid pastry and pies, broil rather than fry, and choose low-fat salad dressings.

8 Avoid long periods of inactivity in front of the television or computer. Move about regularly and use television commercial breaks to walk up and down the stairs a few times to get the body moving again.

9 Shape up with a friend or partner for mutual support (and someone to be active with).

10 If you have a bad day, put it to one side as a single bad day—don't allow it to break your motivation. Go to bed, get up, and start again.

FOOD LABELS

Check food labels for their fat and calorie content. Anything with a total fat content of less than 3 g per 100 g is a low-fat food and is likely to be lower in calories as well. A food with more than 20 g of fat per 100 g is a high-fat food with a high calorie content to match. Compare different brands of the same food for calories, fat, and sodium content— often one brand will be a much better choice.

Change your eating habits

You will find it easier to make lots of small changes rather than big dramatic ones to your eating and drinking habits and they will quickly add up to make a difference. Take a careful look at your habits and pick one or two things that you could start changing today. Then next week pick one or two more changes and make those. At the same time try to add a little more activity every day and you should soon start to see a difference to your body weight and shape, as you trim down and tone up.

Preventing weight gain

Even if not actually overweight, most of us still have to watch what we eat in order to avoid expansion of the waistline. On average many of us finish the year heavier than when we started it. Even if our "food versus energy" balance is out by just 100 calories each day, cumulatively this equates to a weight gain of 8–10 pounds over the year. The amount of food that 100 calories equates to is tiny, for example one small banana, one chocolate cookie, or just ¾ ounce of chips. The rate at which we burn calories depends on our age, gender, size, and degree of fitness. For a 40-year-old moderately sedentary female of 5 ft. 5 in. height and weighing 175 pounds, each of the activities listed on the right would burn 100 calories.

The simple truth is that there are two choices to stop weight gain in its tracks—eat a bit less every day or skip that occasional treat and get more active. The latter will not only help burn calories, but also help relieve stress, boost your immune system, and lower your blood pressure as well.

Easy ways to burn 100 calories …

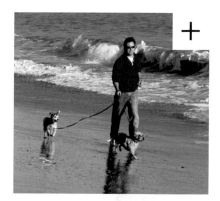 +

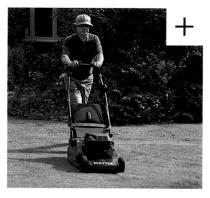 +

+ 15 minutes mowing the lawn
+ 20 minutes weeding the garden
+ 20 minutes walking (moderate)
+ 30 minutes vacuuming/ dusting/mopping floors
+ 30 minutes cleaning windows
+ 30 minutes washing the car
+ 30 minutes dancing around the house to music

what else can I do?

When your blood pressure is high it is also important to consider changing any other habits that will increase your risk of developing heart disease or stroke. For example, if you smoke, stop. Although smoking has little direct effect on blood pressure and giving up is unlikely to lower blood pressure, stopping smoking is undoubtedly one of the most important things you can do to improve your general health.

Other things you can do include being more active, looking at dietary factors such as your intake of omega-3 fatty acids and caffeine, and considering alternative therapies.

"Being inactive increases blood pressure and being more active will help to bring it down"

Be more active

Being active helps with the "food versus energy" balance, weight control, and stress management. In addition, aerobic types of activity improve general fitness and have direct effects on blood pressure. Several studies have found increased levels of activity help to reduce both systolic and diastolic blood pressure in individuals with high blood pressure. They also show that this effect is quickly lost if the activity stops. In order to gain the best benefit, the activity needs to be aerobic and rhythmic, such as swimming, rather than involving weights or vigorous activity, such as playing squash.

The great news is that the activity does not need to be highly energetic or high impact to take effect. Moderate levels of activity are just as effective provided they are done regularly. Current recommendations are to be active for at least 30–45 minutes on at least three to four days each week, at a level appropriate to your age and fitness. Walking, cycling, and swimming are all great forms of moderate activity for people with high blood pressure, and can easily be built by most people into their daily routine. Even modest activity will help to lower blood pressure by 4–8mmHg.

If you have high blood pressure and you already play a non-strenuous sport then there is no need to stop. If your blood pressure is above 180/110mmHg, or if it is poorly controlled, you should undertake a vigorous sport or one involving heavy weights only once your blood pressure is being treated with medication and has been lowered. If you are starting a new activity it is always wise to start slowly and build it up over a few weeks, especially if you are not used to physical activity.

Monitor your activity

Most of us believe that we are more active and fitter than we really are. So be honest with yourself about your activity levels and whether you really are doing at least 30–45 minutes of continuous activity on most days of the week. Over the next few days keep an activity record of what you do, how hard you work, and how long you keep going. Then make a plan of how you can increase your activity to the level necessary for you to stay in great health.

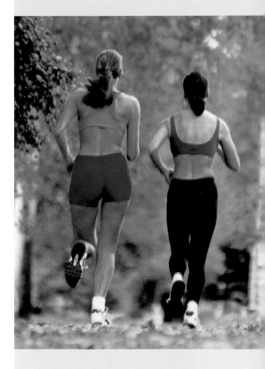

"The European Society for Hypertension (2003) recommends that people with high blood pressure take moderate activity for 30–45 minutes, three to four times each week"

Easy ways to boost your intake of Omega-3 …

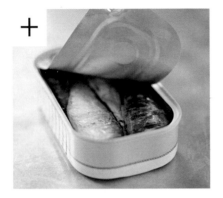

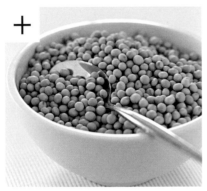

+ Fresh or canned oily fish such as mackerel, herring, salmon, trout, tuna, smelt, pilchards, and sardines
+ Tofu, soybeans, walnuts, walnut oil, sunflower seeds, sesame seeds, pumpkin seeds, and linseeds

Omega-3 fatty acids

Some substances in foods, such as the Omega-3 fatty acids found in fish oils, tend to lower blood pressure. This is because these fatty acids influence the body's production of substances that help the blood vessels to both contract and relax. However, the intake of fish oils required to gain a substantial benefit is large and unlikely to be acquired from diet alone—special fish oil supplements may be prescribed for this effect. The benefits of eating oily fish in terms of maintaining a healthy heart are clearly established, and the recommendation to incorporate two portions of oily fish, such as mackerel, salmon, or tuna, each week into a healthy diet is a good one to follow.

Caffeine

Caffeine is a stimulant, which is generally accepted to increase both blood pressure and heart rate a little. What is less clear is the amount of caffeine likely to have harmful effects, either among people with normal blood pressure or those with high blood pressure. Large doses of caffeine have been shown to increase blood pressure for around four hours after its consumption. However, the doses used in the trials have usually been considerably higher than the 70–80 mg caffeine found in an average cup of coffee.

Moderation appears to be the key here. Drinking four to six cups of coffee each day is unlikely to be harmful. Drinking double espressos could increase blood pressure, as could consuming foods and drinks with added caffeine or the herb guarana. Remember that other drinks contain caffeine as well, including coca cola and hot chocolate, so don't drink too much of these either.

Alternative therapies

Several research studies have shown reductions to blood pressure following massage. A massage appears to help lower both heart rate and blood pressure, and reduces stress and anxiety. In the case of reflexology, little research has been carried out, although high success rates are claimed in treating stress, headaches, and insomnia. If you enjoy alternative treatments and find they help you to relax then go ahead, but remember to tell your therapist about your high blood pressure as this may make a difference to the techniques that they use.

Herbal remedies are also becoming increasingly popular, but as yet little is known about their clinical effectiveness. Those most commonly used for high blood pressure include valerian, hawthorn, and gingko biloba. However, adverse interactions between herbal remedies and medication are not uncommon. It is therefore important that if you are taking prescribed medication always speak to your doctor or pharmacist before you take any herbal supplement. Do not use herbal or alternative therapies as a substitute for conventional treatment (diet, exercise, and medicine).

"It is generally agreed that caffeine increases both blood pressure and heart rate, although it is thought that consuming it in moderation is unlikely to have harmful effects"

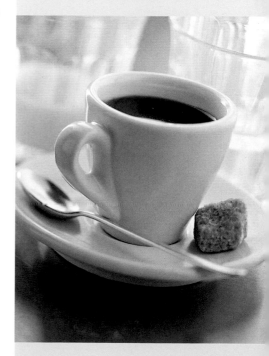

healthy eating plan

	food group	how often?
+	Vegetables, salads, and fruit	Eat plenty every day, aiming for at least five portions, but preferably more
+	Meats, fish, and alternatives	Eat small portions—include oily fish once or twice a week
+	Nuts, seeds, and dried beans	Eat several times a week

examples	why include these?
Artichokes, arugula, broccoli, Brussels sprouts, cabbage, carrots, corn, green beans, kale, leeks, lettuce, mangetout, peas, snow peas, spinach, sweet potatoes, tomatoes, turnips. Apricots, avocados, bananas, blackberries, blueberries, dates, fruit juice or smoothies, grapefruit, grapes, mangoes, melons, oranges, peaches, pears, pineapple, prunes, raisins, raspberries, strawberries, tangerines	Rich sources of vitamins, potassium, fiber, and antioxidants
Select the leanest meat you can afford, trim away any visible fat and broil or roast, instead of frying. Remove skin from poultry, choose all types of fish and include oily fish often (e.g., mackerel, herring, trout, salmon). Quorn or tofu are good alternatives to meat	Rich sources of protein. Oily fish are good sources of Omega-3 essential fatty acids
Almonds, mixed nuts, peanuts, walnuts, sunflower, or pumpkin seeds, kidney beans, lentils, low-salt baked beans, chickpeas, etc.	Rich sources of energy, potassium, protein, and fiber

healthy eating plan

	food group	how often?
+	Starchy and cereal foods	Include these in every meal
+	Low-fat dairy foods	Eat three servings a day
+	Fats and oils	Use in small amounts
+	Sugar and sweet treats	Eat in moderation

examples	why include these?
Bagel, bread (all types but preferably whole wheat, multigrain, or seeded), breakfast cereals (preferably whole wheat), crackers, oats, pasta, potatoes, rice, unsalted popcorn	Major sources of energy and fiber. Add bulk to the diet, keeping you feeling full and satisfied. Buy versions with less than 0.2 g sodium per 100 g
Skim or low-fat milk, fat-free or low-fat yogurt, low-fat cheeses, low-fat custard	Major sources of protein
Choose spreads and oils labeled "polyunsaturated" or "monounsaturated." Olive, walnut, and sesame seed oils are all great choices being rich in monounsaturates. Choose low-fat mayonnaise, light or fat-free salad dressings	Choosing fat wisely and using it sparingly will help with weight management and help keep cholesterol levels in check
Sugar, jelly, jam, and candy, chocolate (choose darker types), fruit concentrates and soft drinks, chewing gum. Cakes, cookies, pies, and pastries are high in fat and so should be treats only	Sugar and sweet treats have no direct effect on blood pressure but will affect weight. Confectionery should be low in fat

menu plans

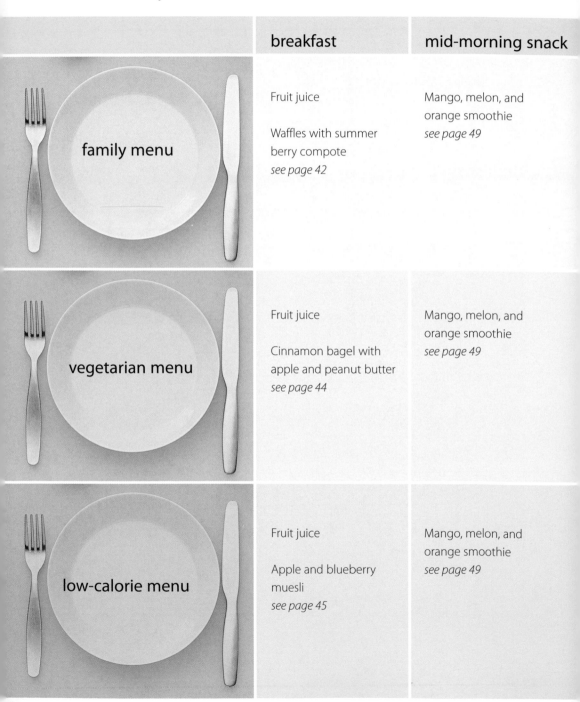

	breakfast	mid-morning snack
family menu	Fruit juice Waffles with summer berry compote *see page 42*	Mango, melon, and orange smoothie *see page 49*
vegetarian menu	Fruit juice Cinnamon bagel with apple and peanut butter *see page 44*	Mango, melon, and orange smoothie *see page 49*
low-calorie menu	Fruit juice Apple and blueberry muesli *see page 45*	Mango, melon, and orange smoothie *see page 49*

lunch	snack	evening meal
Chicken fajitas *see page 52* Tropical fruit salad with ginger and lemongrass syrup *see page 108*	Slice of Banana and pecan teabread *see page 121*	Chicken with lemon and butternut squash *see page 88* Rhubarb and strawberry crumble *see page 112*
Spring vegetable and herb frittata with mixed green salad *see page 63* Low-fat yogurt	Sticky fruit and nut bars *see page 118*	Mushroom stroganoff *see page 95* Tropical fruit salad with ginger and lemongrass syrup *see page 108*
Gazpacho *see page 55* Thai beef salad *see page 64* Low-fat yogurt		Pork escalopes with lemon and caper sauce *see page 81* Caramelized pineapple with apricot coulis *see page 114*

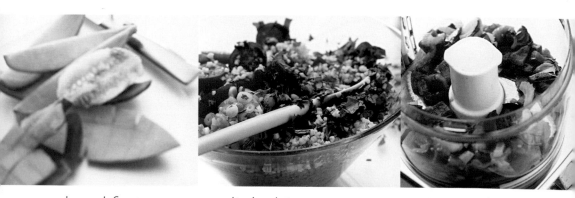

breakfast   light bites   main meals

recipes

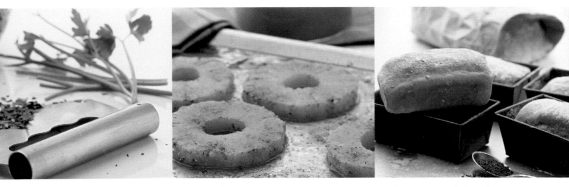

vegetarian   desserts   cakes and bakes

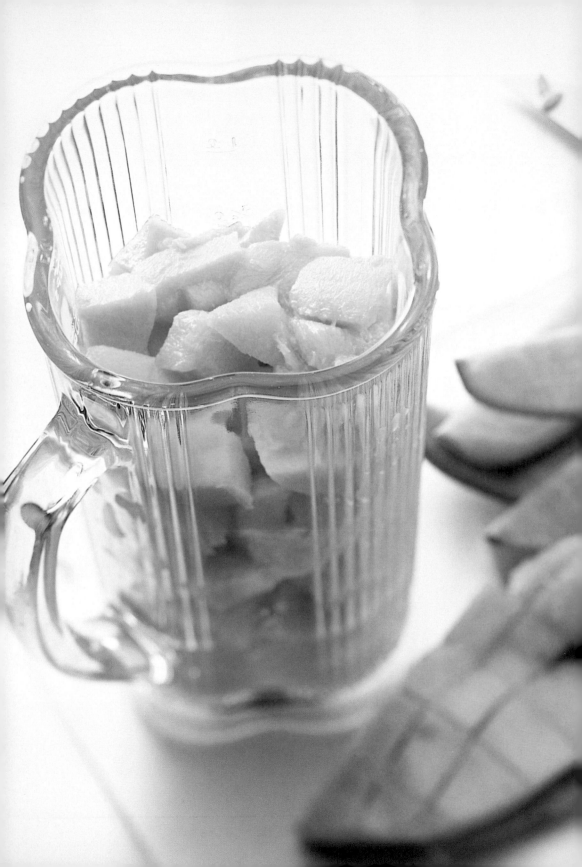

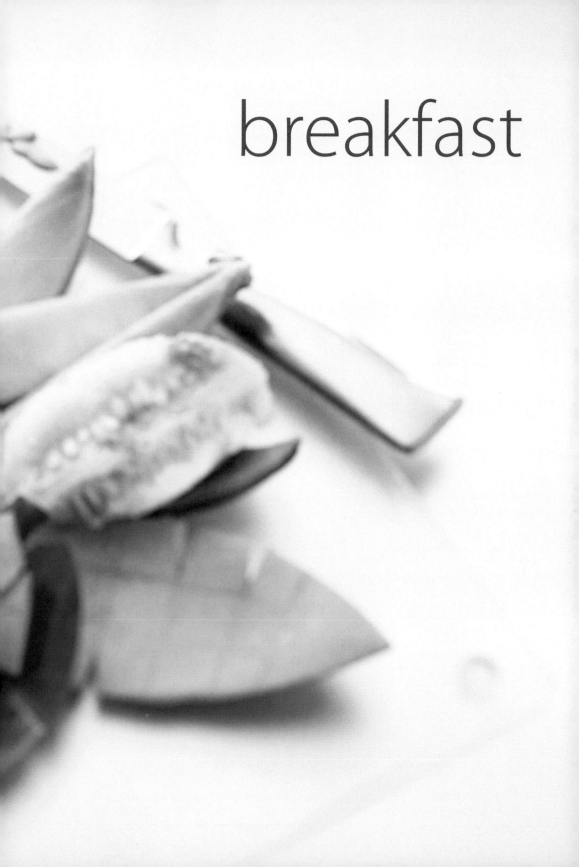

breakfast

Nutritional values

Kcals 410 (1720 Kj)

fat 21 g

saturated fat 12 g

sodium 237 mg

fiber 6 g

Preparation time

5 minutes

Cooking time

5 minutes each waffle

Serves

4

waffles with summer berry compote

½ **cup quartered strawberries**

1¼ **cups raspberries**

¾ **cup blueberries**

2 **tablespoons elderflower cordial**

4 **tablespoons low-fat plain yogurt, to serve**

WAFFLES
⅓ **cup unsalted butter**

½ **cup low-fat milk**

2 **eggs**

1 **cup self-rising whole wheat flour**

3 **tablespoons confectioners' sugar, sifted**

grated zest of ½ **lemon**

1 To make the waffles, first melt the butter, then allow it to cool a little.

2 Pour the milk into a bowl. Separate the eggs then add the yolks to the milk and beat lightly. Add 1 tablespoon of the melted butter to the milk and work in lightly with a fork.

3 Heat a waffle iron on the stove or preheat an electric one while you sift the flour into a bowl. Make a well in the center of the flour and gradually beat in the milk and the remaining butter. Beat the egg whites until stiff enough to hold firm peaks, then fold into the batter with 2 tablespoons of the confectioners' sugar and the lemon zest.

4 Grease the waffle iron and pour in about one eighth of the batter. Close the lid and cook for 4–5 minutes, turning the iron once or twice if using a stove-top model. When the waffle is golden brown and cooked, cover and keep warm while you cook the remaining waffles.

5 Place all the berries and the elderflower cordial in a small saucepan and heat gently until the berries are just starting to release their juice.

6 Put 2 waffles on each plate and serve with the berries and a spoonful of yogurt.

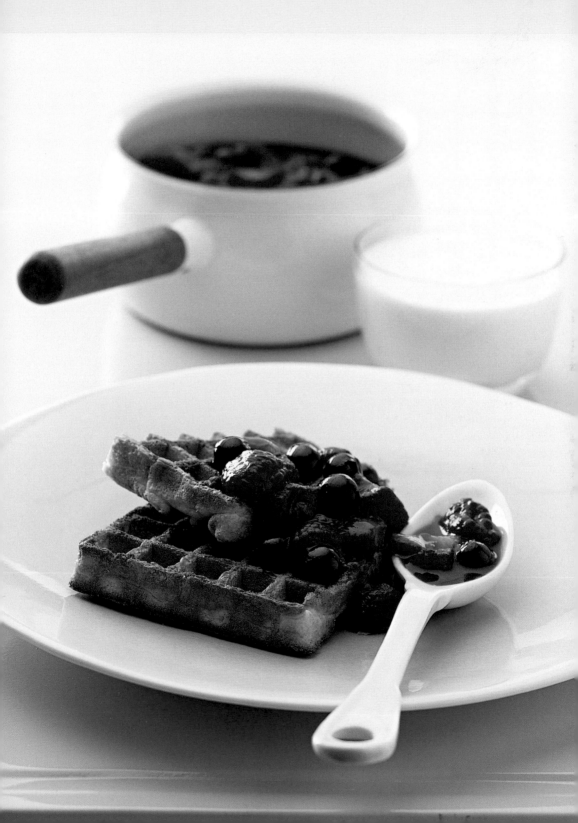

Nutritional values
Kcals 416 (1750 Kj)
fat 14 g
saturated fat 23 g
sodium 470 mg
fiber 4 g

Preparation time
5 minutes
Cooking time
2 minutes
Serves
1

 NUTRITIONAL TIP
Bagels are a low-fat, yet filling, food and make an ideal start to the day when teamed with nutrient-rich raw apple and protein-rich peanut butter to give you lots of energy.

cinnamon bagel with apple and peanut butter

1 crisp dessert apple, grated coarsely

1 heaped tablespoon low-salt smooth peanut butter

1 cinnamon bagel, toasted lightly

1 Stir the grated apple into the peanut butter. Spread the mixture over the bagel and serve immediately.

Nutritional values

Kcals 350 (1479 Kj)

fat 13 g

saturated fat 2 g

sodium 102 mg

fiber 9 g

Preparation time

5 minutes, plus

overnight soaking

Serves

2

apple and blueberry muesli

1 teaspoon raw brown sugar
(optional)

1 apple, peeled and grated
coarsely

½ cup blueberries or
blackberries

⅔ cup low-fat milk

2 tablespoons low-fat plain
yogurt, to serve

SUGAR-FREE MUESLI
¾ cup rolled jumbo oats

1 tablespoon golden raisins
or raisins

1 tablespoon pumpkin or
sunflower seeds

1 tablespoon chopped
almonds

2 tablespoons chopped
ready-to-eat dried apricots

1 Mix all the ingredients for the muesli and store in an
airtight container.

2 To serve, stir in the sugar, if using, the grated apple and
blueberries or blackberries. Divide between two bowls,
pour over the milk, add a spoonful of yogurt, and serve
immediately.

Nutritional values

Kcals 203 (854 Kj)

fat 9 g

saturated fat 1 g

sodium 178 mg

fiber 3 g

Preparation time

15 minutes

Cooking time

25–30 minutes

Makes

12

 NUTRITIONAL TIP

Low-sodium baking powder is available in some health food shops: using this in place of normal baking powder would lower the sodium level considerably.

apple and blackberry muffins

6 tablespoons light brown sugar

1 red apple, about 5 ounces, cored and diced

1 ½ cups blackberries, chopped roughly

1 teaspoon ground cinnamon

2 cups all-purpose whole wheat flour

4 teaspoons baking powder

2 eggs, beaten

½ cup low-fat milk

½ cup canola oil

1 Line a 12-hole muffin pan with paper muffin cases or grease the pan well. Begin by mixing together the sugar, diced apple, blackberries, and cinnamon.

2 Place the flour and baking powder in a bowl, mix together, and make a well in the center. In a separate bowl mix together the eggs, milk, and oil.

3 Pour the liquid into the flour and stir until just blended. Stir in the fruit mixture, taking care not to overmix.

4 Divide the mixture among the muffin cases then bake the muffins in a preheated oven, 400° F., for 20–30 minutes or until a skewer inserted into the center comes out clean. Transfer the muffins to a wire rack to cool.

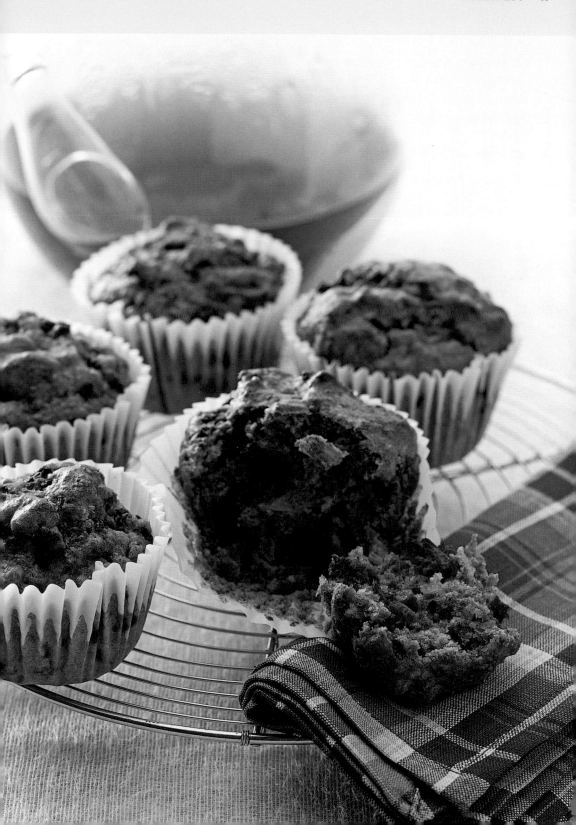

Nutritional values
Kcals 83 (354 Kj)
fat 0.3 g
saturated fat 0 g
sodium 12 mg
fiber 6 g

Preparation time
5 minutes,
plus overnight soaking
Serves
4

autumn fruit compote
with star anise

5 ounces ready-to-eat dried
fruits (such as apricots, apples,
prunes)

2 star anise

¾ cup boiling water

1¼ cups orange juice

Low-fat plain yogurt, to serve

1 Place the dried fruits and star anise in a large heatproof
bowl. Pour over the boiling water, add the orange juice, and
allow to soak overnight at room temperature. Serve with a
spoonful of yogurt.

Nutritional values

Kcals 194 (827 Kj)

fat 0.8 g

saturated fat 0 g

sodium 70 mg

fiber 6 g

Preparation time

5 minutes

Serves

1

NUTRITIONAL TIP

Melons and orange juice contain particularly high amounts of potassium, which helps lower blood pressure, and mango is rich in beta-carotene—one of the antioxidants that helps prevent stroke.

mango, melon, and orange smoothie

1 ripe mango, peeled, seed removed, and chopped roughly

½ galia melon, peeled, seeded, and chopped roughly

¾ cup orange juice

1 Place the mango and melon flesh in a blender. Add the orange juice and blend until smooth. Serve immediately.

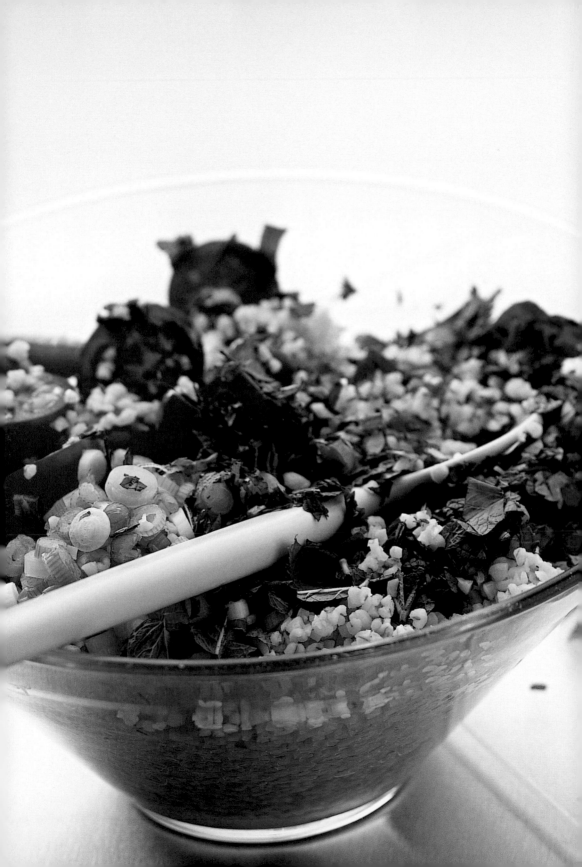

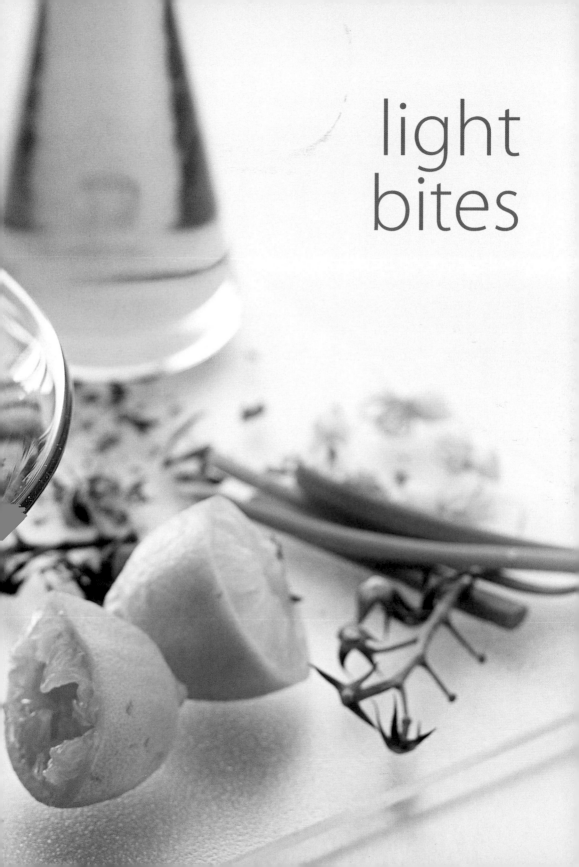

light
bites

Nutritional values
Kcals 332 (1400 Kj)
fat 8 g
saturated fat 2 g
sodium 208 mg
fiber 6 g

Preparation time
15 minutes, plus chiling
Cooking time
10 minutes
Serves
4

chicken fajitas

1 tablespoon olive oil

1 large red onion, sliced thinly

1 red bell pepper, cored, seeded, and sliced thinly

1 yellow bell pepper, cored, seeded, and sliced thinly

14$\frac{1}{2}$ ounces skinned chicken breasts, sliced into thin strips

$\frac{1}{8}$ teaspoon paprika

$\frac{1}{8}$ teaspoon mild chili powder

$\frac{1}{8}$ teaspoon cumin

$\frac{1}{4}$ teaspoon oregano

4 soft flour tortillas

$\frac{1}{2}$ iceberg lettuce, shredded finely

guacamole, to serve (optional)

TOMATO SALSA
1 small red onion, chopped finely

14 ounces small vine-ripened tomatoes

2 garlic cloves, crushed

large handful of fresh cilantro leaves, chopped

freshly ground black pepper

1 First make the tomato salsa. Combine the red onion, tomatoes, garlic, and cilantro leaves in a bowl. Season with black pepper, then cover and chill for 30 minutes to allow the flavors to develop.

2 Heat the oil in a wok or large nonstick skillet. Add the onion and bell peppers and stir-fry for 3–4 minutes. Add the chicken, paprika, chili powder, cumin, and oregano and continue to cook for an additional 5 minutes, or until the chicken is cooked through.

3 Meanwhile, wrap the tortillas in foil and warm in the oven for 5 minutes or according to package instructions.

4 Spoon one quarter of the chicken mixture into the center of each tortilla, add a couple of tablespoons of tomato salsa and the shredded lettuce. Roll up and serve warm, accompanied by guacamole, if desired.

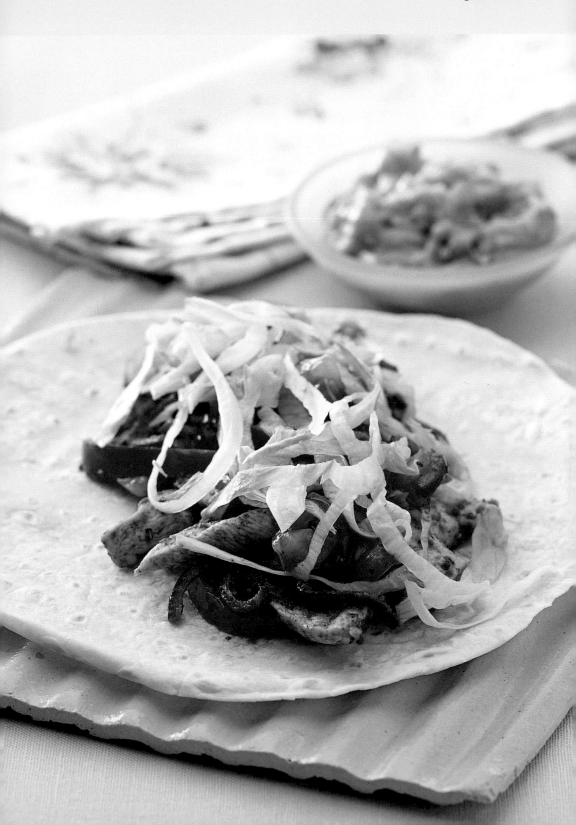

Nutritional values

Kcals 190 (795 Kj)

fat 17 g

saturated fat 3 g

sodium 7 mg

fiber 4 g

Preparation time

10 minutes

Cooking time

40 minutes

Serves

4

NUTRITIONAL TIP

This dip is a healthy treat thanks to the rich potassium content of eggplants and the essential fatty acids in the tahini (a paste made from ground sesame seeds, which is available in health food stores and some supermarkets), all of which help reduce high blood pressure.

baba ghanoush

2 large eggplants, about
1½ pounds total weight

2 fat garlic cloves, crushed

2 tablespoons reduced-salt
tahini

3 tablespoons olive oil

grated zest and juice of
½ lemon

3 tablespoons chopped fresh
cilantro

½ teaspoon smoked paprika

toasted whole wheat pita
bread, to serve

1 Pierce the eggplants several times with a small sharp knife. Place on a baking sheet and cook in a preheated oven, 400° F., for about 40 minutes, or until they feel soft and the skins are beginning to char. Allow to cool.

2 Slice the eggplants in half, scoop out the flesh, and place in a food processor or blender. Add the garlic, tahini, olive oil, lemon zest and juice, and blend until smooth. Stir in the fresh cilantro and smoked paprika. Cover and chill until required. Spread over toasted pita bread and serve.

Nutritional values

Kcals 213 (890 Kj)

fat 12 g

saturated fat 2 g

sodium 160 mg

fiber 4 g

Preparation time

15 minutes, plus chiling

Serves

4–6

NUTRITIONAL TIP

Since it is made with raw vegetables, this Spanish soup is packed with healthy ingredients. Tomatoes and bell peppers, for example, are rich in the antioxidant vitamins A, C, and E, which lower the risk of heart disease and help reduce high blood pressure.

gazpacho

1 pound ripe tomatoes

1 cucumber, peeled, seeded, and chopped roughly

1 red bell pepper, cored, seeded, and chopped

1 small red onion, chopped roughly

1 red chile, seeded, and chopped roughly

3 garlic cloves, chopped roughly

1 cup fresh white breadcrumbs

1 tablespoon tomato paste

1 teaspoon sugar

3 tablespoons red wine vinegar

4 tablespoons olive oil

handful of basil leaves

1¼ cups water

freshly ground black pepper

finely diced cucumber, red bell pepper, and mild onion, to serve

1 Place the tomatoes in a large heatproof bowl and cover with boiling water. Allow to stand for 2 minutes then drain and refresh under cold running water. Peel away the skins, remove the seeds, and roughly chop the flesh.

2 Place the tomato flesh in a food processor or blender with all the other ingredients and process until smooth—you may need to do this in batches. Season with black pepper and chill for at least 1 hour.

3 Ladle the chilled soup into bowls and garnish with finely diced cucumber, red bell pepper, and onion.

Nutritional values

Kcals 134 (563 Kj)

fat 1 g

saturated fat 0.2 g

sodium 528 mg

fiber 2 g

Preparation time

10 minutes, plus

making the stock

Cooking time

10 minutes

Serves

4

NUTRITIONAL TIP

Rinse cooked shrimp thoroughly to reduce their salt content. Vegetable stock can also be used in this recipe: you will need 5 cups. Always look for low-sodium stock when shopping or make your own (see page 102).

hot and sour soup

4 lime leaves

4 slices of fresh ginger root

1 red chile, seeded and sliced

1 lemongrass stalk

1½ cups sliced mushrooms

3½ ounces rice noodles

2 cups baby spinach

4 ounces cooked peeled jumbo shrimp

2 tablespoons lemon juice

freshly ground black pepper

FISH STOCK

2 tablespoons unsalted butter

3 scallions, chopped roughly

1 small leek, chopped roughly

1 celery stick, chopped

2 pounds white fish bones and trimmings

²/₃ cup dry white wine

several parsley stalks

½ lemon, sliced

1 teaspoon black peppercorns

5 cups cold water

1 First make the stock. Melt the butter in a large heavy saucepan, add the vegetables, and fry gently for 5 minutes to soften slightly, without browning. Add the fish bones and trimmings, wine, parsley, lemon slices, peppercorns, and water and bring slowly to a boil. Reduce the heat and simmer for 20 minutes, skimming occasionally. Strain the stock and allow to cool, then chill. Remove any fat from the surface before using.

2 Put the stock, lime leaves, fresh ginger root, chile, and lemongrass in a large saucepan. Cover and bring to a boil. Add the mushrooms and simmer for 2 minutes. Break the noodles into short lengths, drop into the soup, and simmer for 3 minutes.

3 Add the baby spinach and shrimp and simmer for 2 minutes until the shrimp are heated through. Add the lemon juice. Remove and discard the lemongrass stalk and season with black pepper before serving.

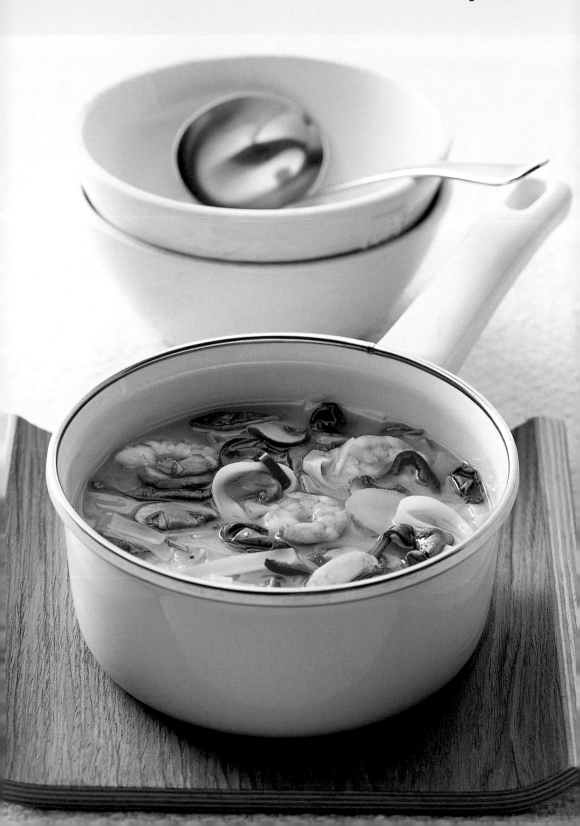

Nutritional values

Kcals 235 (996 Kj)

fat 8 g

saturated fat 1 g

sodium 245 mg

fiber 3 g

Preparation time

15 minutes

Cooking time

5 minutes

Serves

4–6

seared scallops in a spicy dressing

20 large shelled scallops

2 tablespoons sesame oil

12 ounces stir-fry vegetables, such as baby corn, carrot, scallions, sugar snap peas, beansprouts, bok choy, and red bell peppers, all chopped finely

DRESSING
juice of 3 limes

1 tablespoon honey

1 tablespoon rice wine vinegar

1 red chile, seeded and chopped finely

1 To make the dressing, mix together the lime juice, honey, vinegar, and chile.

2 Brush the scallops with a little of the sesame oil. Place on a preheated hot griddle and sear for 2 minutes on each side.

3 Heat the remaining oil in a wok or skillet, add the prepared vegetables, and stir-fry for 2–3 minutes.

4 Spoon the vegetables onto 4 plates, place the scallops on top, and drizzle over the dressing.

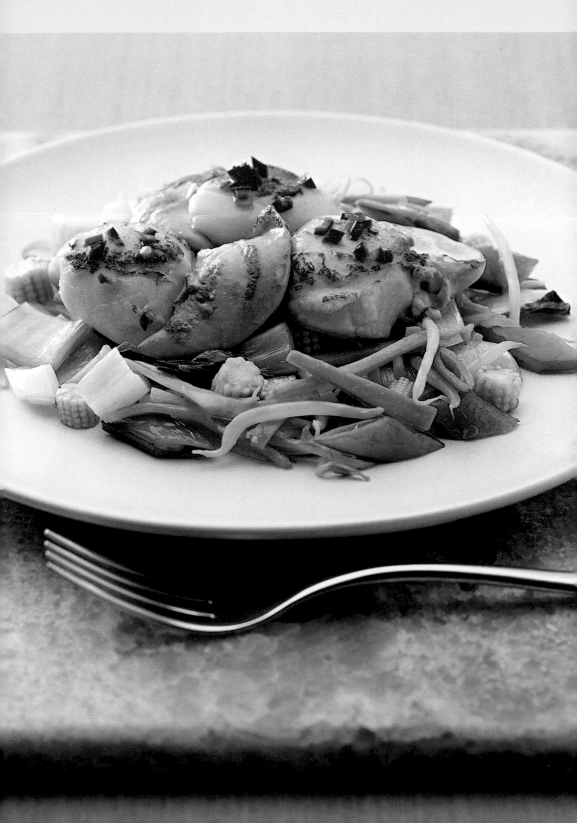

Nutritional values

Kcals 270 (1128 Kj)

fat 9 g

saturated fat 1 g

sodium 12 mg

fiber 1 g

Preparation time

5 minutes, plus standing

Serves

4

NUTRITIONAL TIP

A good way to avoid the need for salt is to use lots of strong flavors. This recipe relies on fresh herbs, garlic, black pepper, and lemon juice for flavor instead of salt.

tabbouleh

1¼ cups bulghur wheat

4 scallions, chopped finely

4 tablespoons chopped mint

4 tablespoons chopped parsley

1 garlic clove, crushed

3 tablespoons olive oil

4 tablespoons lemon juice

10 ounces baby cherry tomatoes, halved

freshly ground black pepper

1 Place the bulghur wheat in a large heatproof bowl, cover with plenty of boiling water and allow to stand for 30 minutes. Drain well.

2 Stir in the scallions, herbs, crushed garlic, olive oil, lemon juice, and tomatoes. Season with black pepper to taste and serve.

Nutritional values
Kcals 605 (2545 Kj)
fat 24 g
saturated fat 3 g
sodium 840 mg
fiber 9 g

Preparation time
20 minutes
Cooking time
40 minutes
Serves
4

coronation chicken salad

1 cup brown rice

6 scallions, chopped finely

4 celery sticks, sliced thinly

1 red bell pepper, cored, seeded, and diced

4 tablespoons reduced-fat mayonnaise

4 tablespoons low-fat plain bio yogurt

2 tablespoons mango chutney

1 tablespoon curry paste

13 ounces cooked chicken breast, skinned and diced

³/₄ cup ready-to-eat dried apricots, sliced thinly

¹/₂ cup slivered almonds, toasted

1 Cook the rice according to the package instructions. Allow to cool then stir in the scallions, celery, and red bell pepper.

2 Mix together the mayonnaise, yogurt, mango chutney, and curry paste in a large bowl.

3 Place the diced chicken and apricots in a separate bowl. Stir in the mayonnaise mixture.

4 Transfer the rice to a serving dish, spoon over the chicken mayonnaise mixture. Garnish with toasted flaked almonds and serve.

Nutritional values
Kcals 288 (1215 Kj)
fat 8 g
saturated fat 2 g
sodium 222 mg
fiber 3 g

Preparation time
10 minutes
Cooking time
10 minutes
Serves
4

✚ NUTRITIONAL TIP
If using canned corn for this recipe, thoroughly rinse it before use to reduce its salt content.

corn and tuna fritters with spicy cucumber salad

1 cup self-rising flour

2 eggs, beaten

²/₃ cup low-fat milk

1 cup corn kernels (cut from 2 ears) or 11-ounce can corn, drained

6¹/₂-ounce can tuna in water, drained and flaked (4 ounces drained weight)

4 scallions, sliced finely

3 tablespoons chopped chives

olive oil, for frying

SALAD
1 small cucumber

2 tablespoons rice wine vinegar

2 tablespoons chili dipping sauce

1 Sift the flour into a large bowl and make a well in the center. Mix together the eggs and milk then gradually beat into the flour to make a smooth batter. Stir in the corn, tuna, scallions, and chives.

2 Heat a little oil in a large nonstick skillet over a medium heat. Cook the fritters in batches. Drop 1 tablespoon of batter into the hot oil and cook for 2 minutes on each side or until golden. Keep the cooked fritters warm on a plate while you cook the remaining fritters in the same way.

3 To make the salad, slice the cucumber in half lengthwise and scoop out and discard the seeds using a small spoon. Cut the cucumber into ¹/₈-inch slices and place in a bowl. Add the rice wine vinegar and chili sauce and mix well. Serve with the cooked fritters.

Nutritional values

Kcals 297 (1235 Kj)

fat 19 g

saturated fat 5 g

sodium 193 mg

fiber 4 g

Preparation time

10 minutes

Cooking time

15 minutes

Serves

4

 NUTRITIONAL TIP

The eggs in this savory omelet are a good source of iron and vitamins. Rich in potassium, the asparagus is also good for controlling blood pressure.

spring vegetable and herb frittata

8 ounces asparagus, chopped into bite-size pieces

1 cup frozen or fresh peas

1 bunch of scallions, sliced thinly

8 large eggs

2 tablespoons low-fat milk

2 tablespoons chopped parsley

2 tablespoons chopped chives

1 tablespoon olive oil

1 Cook the asparagus and peas in a saucepan of boiling water until the asparagus is just tender. Drain well.

2 Beat the eggs with the milk then stir in the drained cooked vegetables and the chopped herbs.

3 Heat the oil in a skillet. Pour in the egg mixture and cook over a medium heat for 5–6 minutes or until the eggs are almost set.

4 Place the skillet under a preheated broiler and cook for an additional 2–3 minutes or until the frittata is brown on top and completely set.

Nutritional values
Kcals 165 (688 Kj)
fat 9 g
saturated fat 2 g
sodium 480 mg
fiber 1 g

Preparation time
15 minutes,
plus standing
Cooking time
12 minutes
Serves
4

thai beef salad

2 x 5-ounce lean sirloin steaks, trimmed

5 ounces baby corn

1 large cucumber

1 small red onion, chopped finely

3 tablespoons chopped fresh cilantro

4 tablespoons rice wine vinegar

4 tablespoons sweet chili dipping sauce

2 tablespoons sesame seeds, lightly toasted

1 Place the steaks on a preheated hot griddle pan and cook for 3–4 minutes on each side. Allow to rest for 10–15 minutes then slice thinly.

2 Place the corn in a saucepan of boiling water and cook for 3–4 minutes or until tender. Refresh under cold water and drain well.

3 Slice the cucumber in half lengthwise then scoop out and discard the seeds using a small spoon. Cut the cucumber into ¼-inch slices.

4 Place the beef, corn, cucumber, red onion, and chopped cilantro in a large bowl. Stir in the rice wine vinegar and chili sauce and mix well. Garnish the salad with sesame seeds and serve.

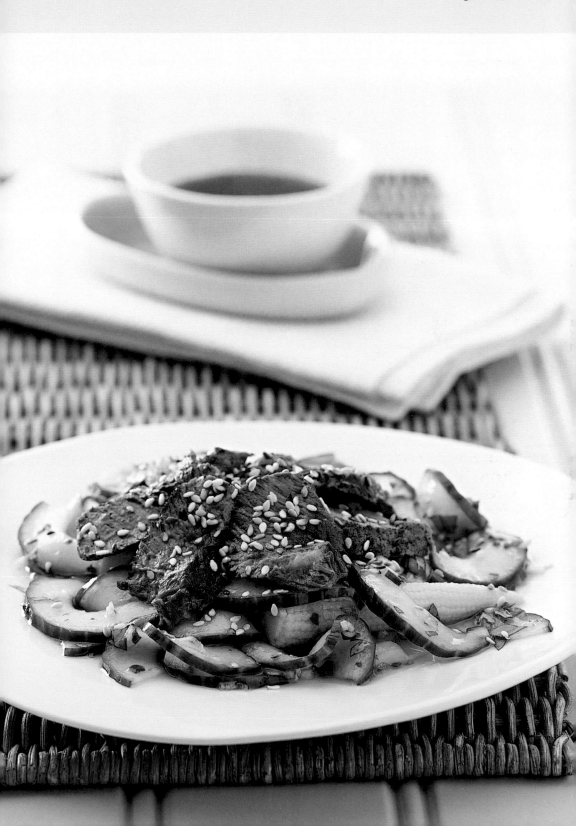

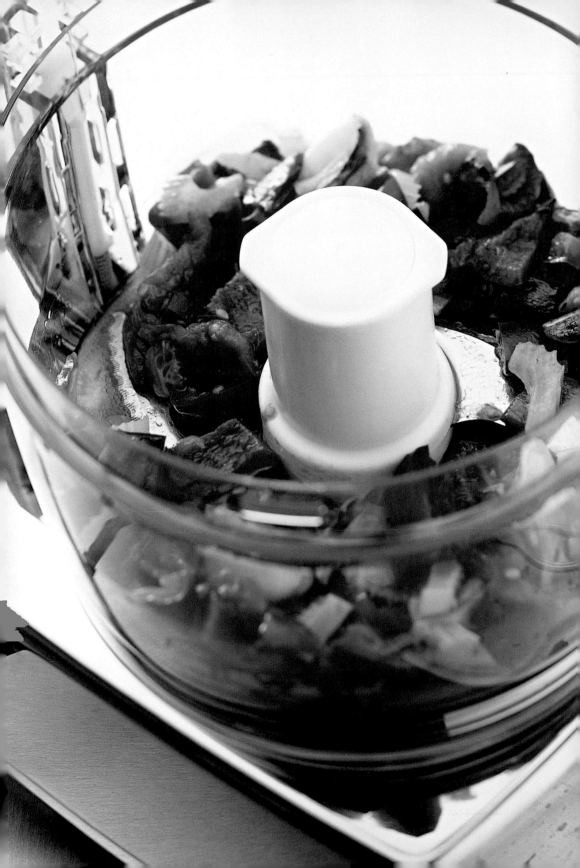

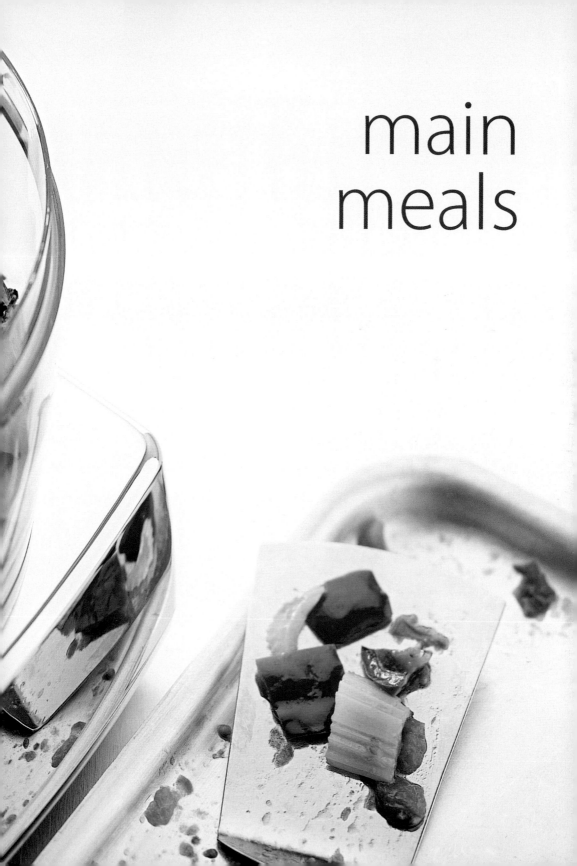

main
meals

Nutritional values

Kcals 374 (1574 Kj)

fat 16 g

saturated fat 3 g

sodium 75 mg

fiber 4 g

Preparation time

10 minutes, plus

cooling

Cooking time

20 minutes

Serves

4

 NUTRITIONAL TIP

Eating oily fish like tuna regularly will ensure your body gets the essential fatty acids it needs for overall health.

seared tuna with mexican salsa

4 tuna steaks, each about 4 ounces

olive oil, for brushing

SALSA
3 corn ears

1 small red onion, chopped finely

1 garlic clove, crushed

1 red bell pepper, cored, seeded, and diced finely

1 red chile, seeded and chopped finely

2 tablespoons extra virgin olive oil

juice of 1 lime

4 tablespoons chopped fresh cilantro

1 To make the salsa, place the corn ears under a preheated hot broiler and cook until golden brown all over. Allow to cool, then remove the kernels from the ears with a sharp knife and mix with the red onion, garlic, red bell pepper, chile, olive oil, and lime juice. Stir in the fresh cilantro. Cover and set aside.

2 Brush the tuna steaks with oil and cook on a preheated hot griddle pan for 4–5 minutes on each side. Serve with the salsa.

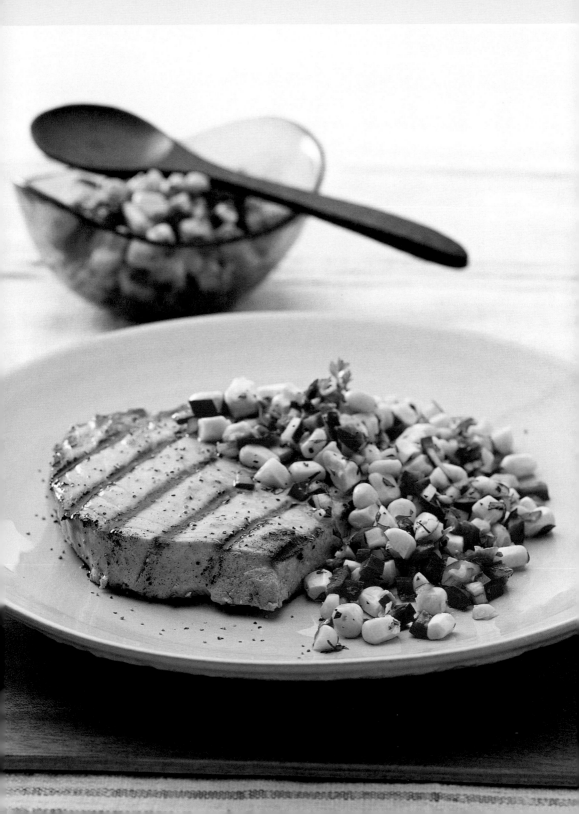

Nutritional values
Kcals 236 (998 Kj)
fat 6 g
saturated fat 3 g
sodium 229 mg
fiber 0 g

Preparation time
5 minutes,
plus marinating
Cooking time
15 minutes
Serves
4

thai spiced cod

4 cod fillets, skin on, each about 7$\frac{1}{2}$ ounces

freshly ground black pepper

jasmine rice, to serve

lime wedges and mint leaves, to garnish

MARINADE
2 large garlic cloves

2 tablespoons chopped fresh cilantro

1 tablespoon chopped mint

$\frac{1}{2}$ green chile, seeded

finely grated zest and juice of 1 lime

1 tablespoon palm sugar or granulated brown sugar

$\frac{3}{4}$ cup reduced-fat coconut milk

1 To make the marinade, place the garlic, cilantro, mint, chile, lime zest and juice, sugar, and coconut milk in a food processor or blender and blend briefly until smooth.

2 Place the cod fillets in a shallow dish, pour over the marinade and leave in a cool place for 1 hour, turning once.

3 Lift the fish out of the marinade and lay the fillets skin-side down on a lightly greased baking sheet. Cook in a preheated oven, 400° F., for 15 minutes.

4 Tip the remaining marinade into a saucepan. Bring to a boil, then reduce the heat and simmer for 1 minute.

5 Place the fish on 4 warm plates, spoon over the marinade and serve with jasmine rice and garnished with lime wedges and mint leaves.

Nutritional values

Kcals 320 (1345 Kj)

fat 11 g

saturated fat 2 g

sodium 678 mg

fiber 5 g

Preparation time

10 minutes

Cooking time

35 minutes

Serves

4

 NUTRITIONAL TIP

Tomatoes are a very good source of potassium, the mineral that helps counteract the effects of salt on blood pressure.

mediterranean fish casserole

2 tablespoons olive oil

2 large garlic cloves, crushed

2 red onions, sliced

2 red bell peppers, cored, seeded, and sliced into thin strips

1 large fennel bulb, sliced thinly

2 x 13-ounce cans chopped tomatoes

1 tablespoon sun-dried tomato paste

4 tablespoons Pernod

1 pound 7 ounces skinless firm white fish fillets (such as cod, haddock, halibut), cut into bite-size pieces

¼ cup pitted black olives, rinsed well and drained

freshly ground black pepper

thyme, to garnish

1 Heat the oil in a shallow flameproof casserole and stir in the garlic and onions. Cover and fry slowly for about 10 minutes or until the onions are beginning to soften. Add the bell peppers and fennel and cook, stirring, for 1 minute.

2 Add the canned tomatoes, tomato paste, Pernod, and black pepper.

3 Bring to a boil, reduce the heat, and simmer, uncovered, for 15 minutes. Stir in the fish and simmer for an additional 3–5 minutes or until the fish is just cooked. Stir in the olives and serve garnished with thyme.

Nutritional values

Kcals 245 (1024 Kj)

fat 15 g

saturated fat 3 g

sodium 203 mg

fiber 0 g

Preparation time

10 minutes,

plus marinating

Cooking time

15 minutes

Serves

4

NUTRITIONAL TIP

Using spices rules out the need for salt in cooking, a good habit to adopt since overuse of salt will adversely affect your blood pressure. Pre-menopausal women and children should not eat swordfish.

moroccan spiced swordfish

3 garlic cloves, chopped finely

½ teaspoon ground cumin

½ teaspoon ground turmeric

¼ teaspoon paprika

¼ teaspoon hot chili powder

grated zest and juice of
1 lemon

3 tablespoons olive oil

3 tablespoons chopped
parsley

3 tablespoons chopped fresh
cilantro

4 swordfish steaks, each about
5 ounces

French beans and reduced-fat
tzatziki, to serve (optional)

1 Combine the garlic, spices, lemon zest and juice, olive oil, and herbs.

2 Place the fish on a lightly oiled baking sheet and top each piece of fish with a thick coating of the spice mixture. Cover loosely with plastic wrap, transfer to the refrigerator, and allow to marinate for 1 hour.

3 Remove the plastic wrap then bake the fish in a preheated oven, 350° F., for 15 minutes or until it begins to turn opaque. Serve with French beans and tzatziki, if desired.

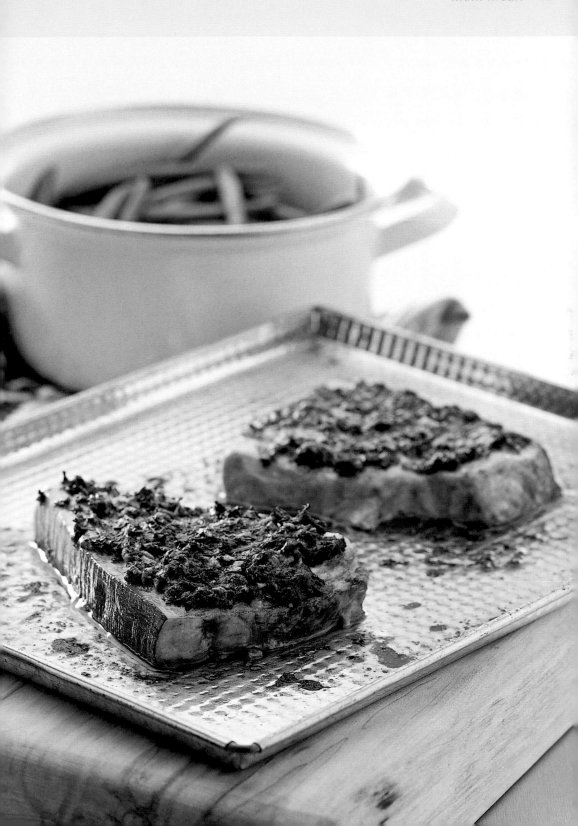

Nutritional values

Kcals 328 (1365 Kj)

fat 20 g

saturated fat 4 g

sodium 149 mg

fiber 2 g

Preparation time

5 minutes

Cooking time

10 minutes

Serves

4

maple and mustard glazed salmon

2 tablespoons low-salt wholegrain mustard

1 tablespoon maple syrup

4 salmon fillets, skin on, each about 4 ounces

14½ ounces asparagus or tender stem broccoli

1 Mix the mustard with the maple syrup to make a glaze for the salmon.

2 Place the salmon fillets, skin side down, on a shallow ovenproof tray lined with foil and spread the glaze over them. Place under a preheated broiler and cook for 10 minutes, depending on thickness, until cooked through.

3 Meanwhile, steam the asparagus or broccoli until just tender. Transfer to 4 warm plates, top with the salmon and serve with new potatoes.

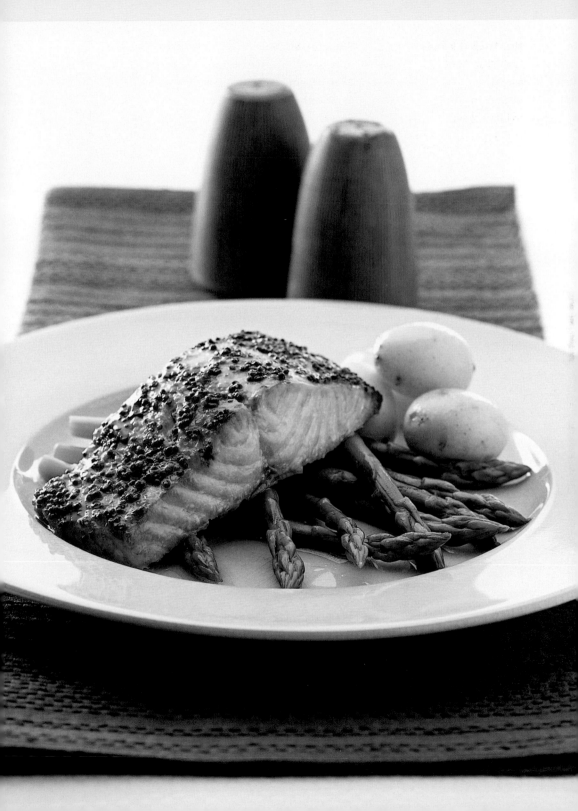

Nutritional values

Kcals 250 (1055 Kj)

fat 10 g

saturated fat 2 g

sodium 211 mg

fiber 3 g

Preparation time

15 minutes

Cooking time

20 minutes

Serves

4

NUTRITIONAL TIP

Both peppers and garlic lower the risk of heart disease and stroke and help reduce high blood pressure. If you buy the fish from a fish merchant they will skin it for you to save you doing it.

flounder with bell pepper sauce

2 red bell peppers, cored, seeded, and chopped roughly

6 plum tomatoes, skinned and chopped roughly

2 celery sticks, chopped roughly

3 fat garlic cloves

1 tablespoon olive oil

8 small flounder fillets, total weight about 1 pound

4 teaspoons pesto

²/₃ cup dry white wine

freshly ground black pepper

tender stem broccoli, to serve (optional)

1 Place the red peppers, tomatoes, celery, and garlic in a large roasting pan, drizzle over the olive oil, and season with black pepper. Cook in a preheated oven, 450° F., for 15–20 minutes, or until the vegetables are soft.

2 Meanwhile, remove the skin from the fish fillets, then lay the fish, skinned side uppermost, on a board. Spread each one with ½ teaspoon pesto and roll up the fillets as you would a jelly roll.

3 Pour the wine into a flameproof casserole dish and add the rolled fish, seam side down. Bring the wine to a boil then cover the pan with a lid or foil, reduce the heat, and leave to simmer for about 10 minutes. Using a slotted spoon, remove the fish and place in a warm serving dish. Reserve the wine.

4 Place the roasted vegetables and the wine in a food processor or blender and blend for 2–3 minutes until smooth. Return to the pan, reheat, and season to taste. Serve as an accompaniment to the fish, with tender stem broccoli, if desired.

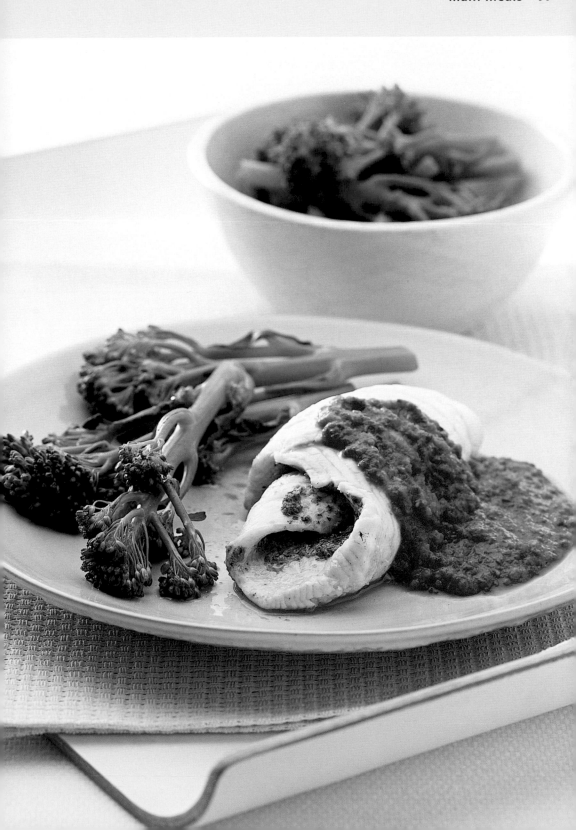

Nutritional values
Kcals 655 (2745 Kj)
fat 32 g
saturated fat 14 g
sodium 136 mg
fiber 7 g

Preparation time
20 minutes
Cooking time
20 minutes
Serves
4

NUTRITIONAL TIP
If the fat is trimmed off the chops before cooking and they are broiled, this dish will contain 12 g less fat, including 5 g less saturated fat, per serving.

lamb with mustard mash
and mushrooms

3 teaspoons olive oil

8 lamb chops, each about 4 ounces

8 ounces mushrooms, quartered

4 tablespoons reduced-sugar cranberry jelly

watercress, to garnish

MUSTARD MASH
3 pounds floury potatoes, peeled and cut into equal-size chunks

½ cup hot low-fat milk

1 tablespoon low-salt wholegrain mustard

small piece of unsalted butter

1 To make the mash, place the potatoes in a large saucepan of boiling water and simmer for 20 minutes or until tender. Drain well and return to the saucepan, add the hot milk, mustard, and butter and mash well.

2 Meanwhile, heat 1 teaspoon of the oil in a nonstick skillet and fry the lamb chops for 3–4 minutes on each side. Remove from the pan and keep warm. Add the remaining oil and cook the mushrooms for 2–3 minutes. Add the cranberry jelly and cook for an additional 2–3 minutes.

3 Spoon the potato onto 4 plates, place the lamb on top of the mash, and pour over the mushrooms and any remaining pan juices. Garnish with watercress and serve.

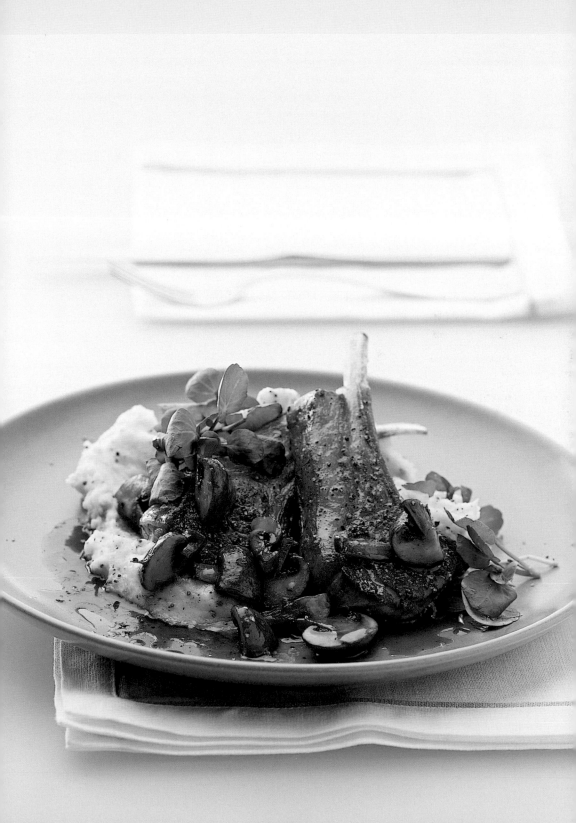

Nutritional values

Kcals 282 (1184 Kj)

fat 14 g

saturated fat 87 g

sodium 159 mg

fiber 1 g

Preparation time

10 minutes,

plus marinating

Cooking time

10–15 minutes

Serves

4

 NUTRITIONAL TIP

Yogurt is the basis for this marinade. It is an excellent source of calcium, which is essential for strong bones and teeth.

lamb marinated in saffron, lemon, and yogurt

pinch of sugar

generous pinch of saffron threads

1 tablespoon hot water

4 tablespoons lemon juice

¼ cup low-fat plain yogurt

1 onion, grated coarsely

¾-inch piece of fresh ginger root, peeled and chopped finely

½ teaspoon cayenne pepper

5 tablespoons roughly chopped fresh cilantro

4 lamb leg steaks, trimmed of fat, each about 4 ounces

freshly ground black pepper

1 Put the sugar and saffron in a mortar and grind to a powder. Add the hot water and set aside.

2 Mix together the lemon juice, yogurt, grated onion, fresh ginger, cayenne pepper, and fresh cilantro. Stir in the saffron liquid.

3 Place the lamb steaks in a large shallow dish. Spoon over the yogurt mixture and make sure the lamb is well coated. Cover and chill for at least 8 hours.

4 Transfer the lamb to a baking sheet covered with foil. Place under a preheated broiler and cook for 5–7 minutes on each side or until cooked to your liking.

Nutritional values

Kcals 345 (1430 Kj)

fat 26 g

saturated fat 6 g

sodium 97 mg

fiber 0 g

Preparation time

15 minutes

Cooking time

10 minutes

Serves

4

pork escalopes with lemon and caper sauce

3 tablespoons chopped Italian parsley

3 tablespoons chopped mint

4–6 tablespoons lemon juice

1 tablespoon capers, drained and rinsed

6 tablespoons olive oil, plus extra for brushing

4 pork escalopes, each about 4 ounces, trimmed

baby new potatoes and steamed asparagus, to serve (optional)

1 Place the herbs, lemon juice, capers, and olive oil in a blender and blend until smooth to make a dressing.

2 Brush the pork with olive oil. Place on a preheated hot griddle pan and cook for 2–3 minutes on each side or until cooked through.

3 Drizzle the herby dressing over the pork. Serve with baby new potatoes and steamed asparagus, if desired.

Nutritional values
Kcals 508 (2130 Kj)
fat 20 g
saturated fat 5 g
sodium 342 mg
fiber 0.5 g

Preparation time
10 minutes
Cooking time
about 20 minutes
Serves
2

duck with cinnamon
and cranberry sauce

2 boneless duck breasts, each about 10 ounces

1 tablespoon olive oil

1 small red onion, chopped finely

1 garlic clove, chopped finely

¾ cup low-sodium chicken bouillon

¾ cup red wine

pinch of ground cinnamon

1 tablespoon reduced-sugar cranberry jelly

freshly ground black pepper

Puy lentils and sugar snap peas, to serve (optional)

1 Place the duck breasts, skin side down, in a hot pan and cook for 2–3 minutes or until brown. Turn them over and brown the other side. (By browning them skin side down first there should be no need to add any fat.)

2 Transfer the duck breasts to a roasting pan and cook in a preheated oven, 400° F., for 15 minutes or until cooked through.

3 While the duck is cooking, heat the oil in a nonstick pan, add the onion and garlic, and cook, stirring occasionally, for about 2–3 minutes. Add the bouillon, red wine, and cinnamon and bring to a boil. Allow the sauce to bubble for about 10 minutes or until reduced by half. Strain the sauce and discard the onion. Season with black pepper and stir in the cranberry jelly.

4 Thickly slice the duck and transfer to 2 warm plates. Spoon over a little of the sauce and serve with Puy lentils and sugar snap peas, if desired.

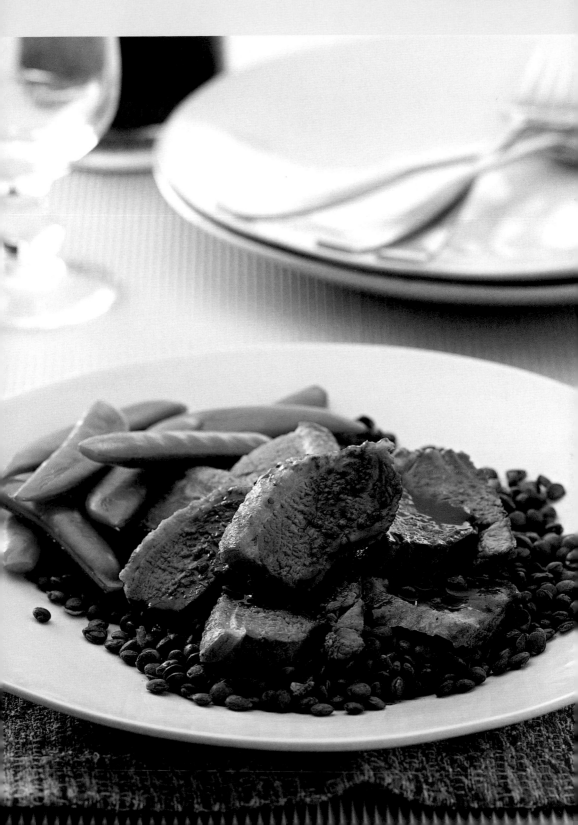

Nutritional values

Kcals 493 (2068 Kj)

fat 16 g

saturated fat 6 g

sodium 347 mg

fiber 2 g

Preparation time

15 minutes

Cooking time

40 minutes

Serves

4

beef ragout with rosemary polenta wedges

1 tablespoon olive oil

1 red onion, chopped finely

1 fat garlic clove, chopped

2 celery sticks, sliced

1 pound lean ground beef

2 x 13-ounce cans chopped tomatoes

¼ cup tomato paste

¾ cup red wine

1 teaspoon dried mixed herbs

freshly ground black pepper

POLENTA
1 cup quick-cook cornmeal

1 cup freshly grated Parmesan cheese

⅓ cup roughly chopped sun-dried tomatoes (not in oil)

2 tablespoons pitted black olives, drained, rinsed, and chopped roughly

1 teaspoon roughly chopped rosemary

1 tablespoon unsalted butter

1 Heat the oil in a large nonstick saucepan. Add the onion, garlic, and celery and cook for 5 minutes or until beginning to soften. Add the ground beef and cook over a medium heat until browned.

2 Stir in the tomatoes, tomato paste, red wine, dried mixed herbs, and black pepper. Bring to a boil then reduce the heat and simmer for 30 minutes or until the liquid is reduced.

3 To make the polenta wedges, pour 2½ cups water into a large saucepan and bring to a boil. Pour in the cornmeal in a slow, steady stream, stirring continuously. Reduce the heat to low and cook for 1 minute or until thick. Stir in the Parmesan, sun-dried tomatoes, olives, rosemary, and butter, and add pepper to taste. Spread the polenta in a lightly oiled, 7 x 11 inch shallow pan. Allow to cool then cut into 8 rectangles. Cut each rectangle in half diagonally to make 16 triangles.

4 Place the polenta under a preheated hot broiler for 3–4 minutes. Transfer to a warm plate and serve with the beef sauce.

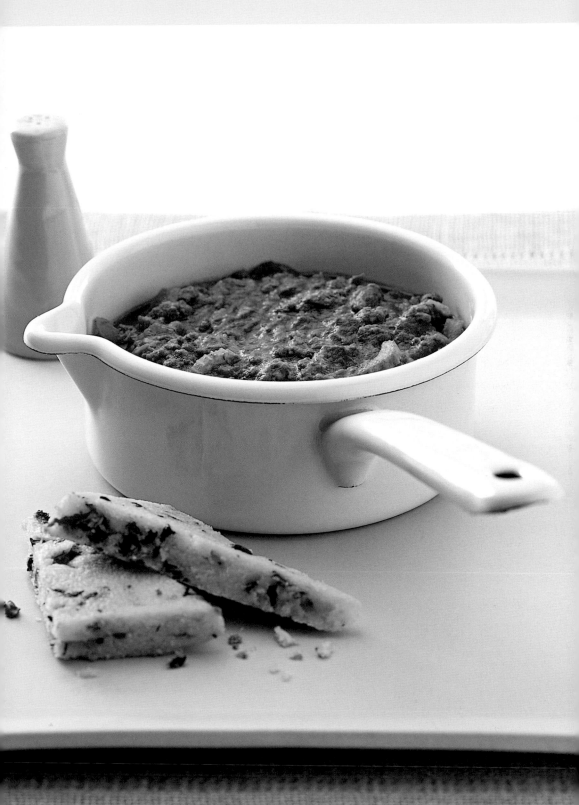

Nutritional values
Kcals 400 (1673 Kj)
fat 24 g
saturated fat 5 g
sodium 79 mg
fiber 2 g

Preparation time
20 minutes,
plus marinating
Cooking time
20 minutes
Serves
4

NUTRITIONAL TIP
Marinating meat or fish in lemon or lime juice before cooking helps avoid the need for salt to add flavor.

beef satay

1 pound sirloin steak, trimmed and sliced into 1-inch thick strips

4 tablespoons lemon juice

1 fat garlic clove, crushed

1 tablespoon granulated brown sugar

1 teaspoon ground cumin

1 teaspoon ground coriander

1 teaspoon finely chopped fresh ginger root

stir-fried vegetables, to serve

SATAY SAUCE
1 tablespoon rapeseed oil

1 small onion, chopped finely

1 fat garlic clove, crushed or chopped finely

6 tablespoons low-salt crunchy peanut butter

1 tablespoon granulated brown sugar

$^1/_2$ teaspoon chili flakes

grated zest and juice of 1 lemon

1 Soak 8 wooden skewers in a bowl of water for 15 minutes. Place the strips of beef between 2 sheets of plastic wrap and beat until thin using a meat mallet or rolling pin. Transfer to a shallow dish. Mix together the lemon juice, garlic, sugar, cumin, ground coriander, and ginger, then pour over the meat. Stir well to coat all the meat, then leave to marinate for 30 minutes.

2 To make the satay sauce, heat the oil in a saucepan and add the onion and garlic. Cook, stirring, for 1–2 minutes. Add the peanut butter, sugar, chili flakes, lemon juice and zest, and $^3/_4$ cup water. Bring to a boil then reduce the heat and cook for 10 minutes or until the sauce begins to thicken.

3 Thread the meat onto the soaked skewers, then place on a preheated hot griddle pan or under the broiler for 3–4 minutes. Turn and cook for an additional 3–4 minutes, or until the meat is cooked.

4 Serve the meat on a bed of stir-fried vegetables, topped with a little satay sauce.

Nutritional values

Kcals 422 (1766 Kj)

fat 18 g

saturated fat 3 g

sodium 126 mg

fiber 4 g

Preparation time

15 minutes

Cooking time

45–50 minutes

Serves

4

chicken with sweet and sour onions

4 skinless chicken breasts

3 tablespoons olive oil

5 red onions, sliced thinly

2 tablespoons balsamic vinegar

1 tablespoon sugar

½ cup raisins

¼ cup pine nuts, lightly toasted

freshly ground black pepper

tender stem broccoli, to serve

1 Using a sharp knife, slice the chicken breasts almost in half lengthwise. Spread each piece of chicken between 2 sheets of waxed paper or plastic wrap and beat with a meat mallet or rolling pin until thin. Lightly brush with a little of the olive oil.

2 Heat the remaining oil in a heavy-based nonstick saucepan. Add the onions and cook over a gentle heat for 30 minutes, stirring occasionally. Add the vinegar, sugar, and raisins and cook for an additional 10 minutes. Season to taste with pepper.

3 Place the chicken on a preheated hot griddle pan and cook for 2–3 minutes on each side.

4 Spoon the onion mixture onto 4 plates, top with the chicken, and sprinkle with the pine nuts. Serve with tender stem broccoli.

Nutritional values
Kcals 336 (1408 Kj)
fat 18 g
saturated fat 4 g
sodium 82 mg
fiber 3 g

Preparation time
10 minutes
Cooking time
30–40 minutes
Serves
4

NUTRITIONAL TIP
Skinning the chicken thighs before cooking them would reduce the amount of fat by 7 g and saturated fat by 2 g.

chicken with lemon and butternut squash

8 chicken thighs, skin on

1 butternut squash, about 2 pounds, peeled, seeded, and cut into large chunks

2 red onions, cut into wedges

8 garlic cloves

2 small lemons

1 tablespoon honey

2 tablespoons olive oil

6 rosemary sprigs

freshly ground black pepper

1 Place the chicken thighs, butternut squash, onion wedges, and 6 of the garlic cloves in a single layer in a large roasting pan (or use 2 medium pans). Grate the zest from 1 lemon and squeeze the juice and set aside. Slice the other into wedges and add to the roasting pan.

2 Crush or finely chop the remaining garlic and mix with the lemon zest and juice, honey, and oil. Pour the mixture over the chicken and vegetables. Sprinkle over the rosemary and season with black pepper.

3 Bake in a preheated oven, 400° F., for about 30–40 minutes, or until the chicken is cooked through.

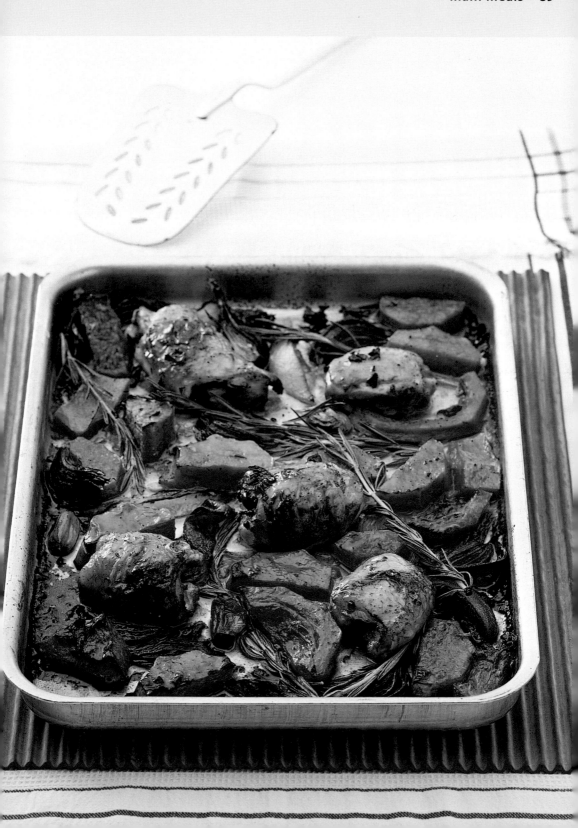

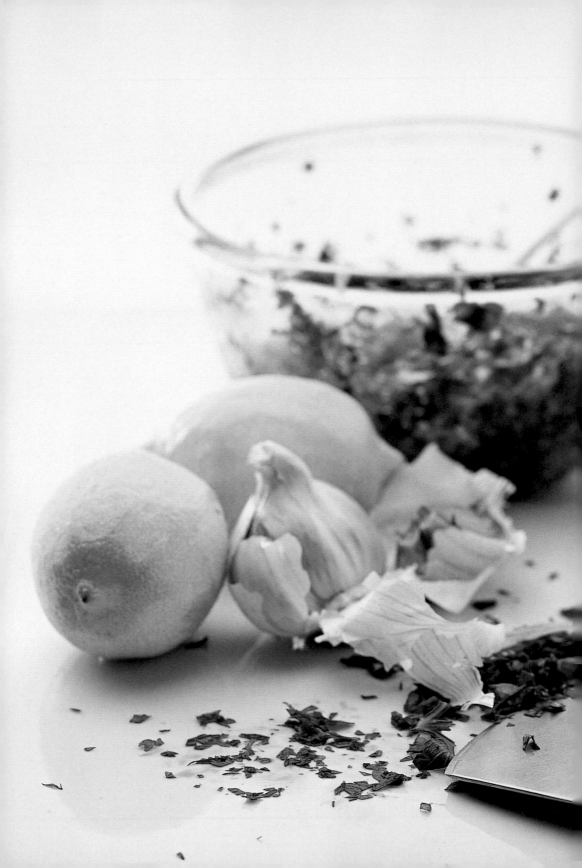

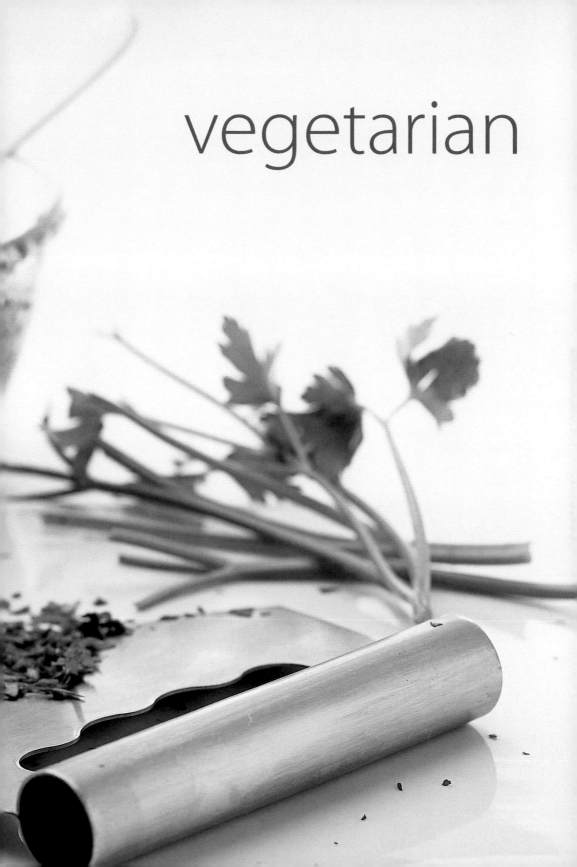

vegetarian

Nutritional values

Kcals 500 (2122 Kj)

fat 11 g

saturated fat 1 g

sodium 9 mg

fiber 6 g

Preparation time

15 minutes

Cooking time

13 minutes

Serves

4

zucchini with linguine
and gremolata

2 tablespoons olive oil

6 large zucchini, sliced thickly

8 scallions, sliced finely

14½ ounces linguine

shavings of fresh Parmesan
cheese, to serve

GREMOLATA
grated zest of 2 unwaxed
lemons

1 tablespoon oil

10 tablespoons chopped
Italian parsley

2 garlic cloves, crushed

1 To make the gremolata, mix the lemon zest and oil with the parsley and garlic.

2 Heat the oil in a nonstick skillet, add the sliced zucchini and cook over a high heat, stirring, for 10 minutes or until brown. Add the scallions and cook for 1–2 minutes.

3 Meanwhile, cook the pasta according to the package instructions. Drain well then stir in the zucchini, scallions, and gremolata. Serve at once, topped with shavings of fresh Parmesan.

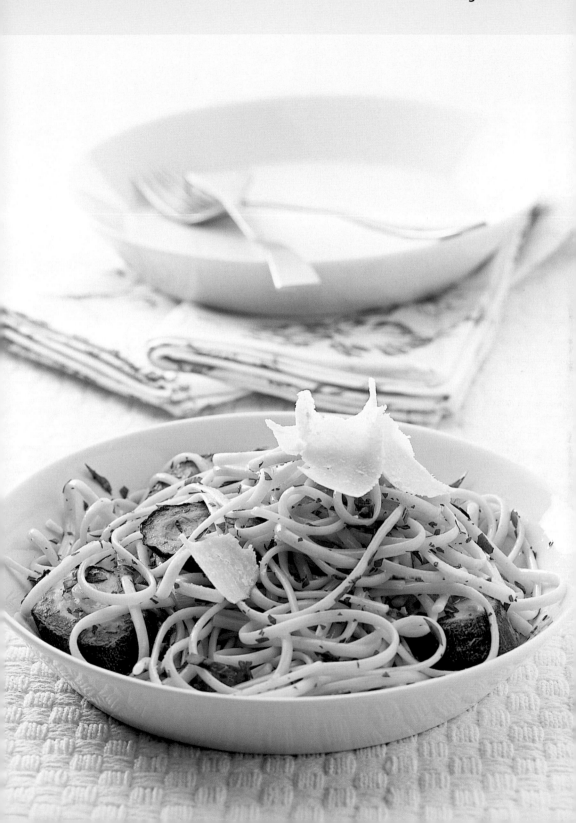

Nutritional values

Kcals 250 (1054 Kj)

fat 10 g

saturated fat 2 g

sodium 472 mg

fiber 3 g

Preparation time

10 minutes

Cooking time

35–40 minutes

Serves

4

butternut squash
and spinach curry

1 tablespoon rapeseed oil

1 large onion, chopped finely

**1 butternut squash or
pumpkin, about 3 pounds,
peeled, seeded, and cut into
large cubes**

**4 tablespoons mild curry
paste**

**1 tablespoon reduced-fat
coconut milk**

**¾ cup low-salt vegetable
stock**

**8 ounces leaf spinach, washed
and chopped roughly**

**½ cup low-fat plain
bio yogurt**

freshly ground black pepper

basmati rice, to serve

1 Heat the oil in a large heavy skillet. Add the onion and cook, stirring, for 2 minutes or until soft. Add the butternut squash or pumpkin and curry paste and continue to cook for 2–3 minutes.

2 Add the coconut milk and vegetable stock and bring to a boil. Cover and simmer over a low heat for 20 minutes.

3 Add the spinach in batches, stirring after each batch, until wilted. Stir in the yogurt and cook for an additional 10 minutes. Season with black pepper and serve with basmati rice.

Nutritional values

Kcals 150 (625 Kj)

fat 11 g

saturated fat 5 g

sodium 43 mg

fiber 5 g

Preparation time

10 minutes

Cooking time

25 minutes

Serves

4

 NUTRITIONAL TIP

Not only is this stroganoff a tasty vegetarian dish, its main ingredient, mushrooms, are a good source of potassium, which has a beneficial effect on blood pressure.

mushroom stroganoff

1 tablespoon rapeseed oil

1 large onion, sliced thinly

4 celery sticks, sliced thinly

2 garlic cloves, crushed

1 pound 3 ounces mixed mushrooms, chopped roughly

2 teaspoons smoked paprika

1 cup low-sodium Vegetable stock (see page 102)

²/₃ cup sour cream

freshly ground black pepper

boiled rice, to serve

1 Heat the oil in a nonstick skillet, add the onion, celery, and garlic and cook for 5 minutes. Add the mushrooms and paprika and cook for another 5 minutes. Pour in the stock and cook for an additional 10 minutes or until the liquid is reduced by half.

2 Stir in the sour cream and black pepper to taste and cook over a medium heat for 5 minutes. Serve at once with boiled rice.

Nutritional values

Kcals 365 (1535 Kj)

fat 14 g

saturated fat 3 g

sodium 566 mg

fiber 12 g

Preparation time

15 minutes, plus

cooling

Cooking time

1–1½ hours

Serves

4

chickpea salad

1½ cups dried chickpeas, soaked overnight in cold water

13 ounces cherry tomatoes, halved

4 celery sticks, sliced

2 ounces Kalamata olives, whole, rinsed well, and drained

4 scallions, chopped finely

Mint and yogurt dressing (see page 98)

freshly ground black pepper

mint leaves, to garnish

1 Drain the chickpeas, rinse well, and drain again. Put them into a large saucepan, cover with plenty of cold water and bring to a boil. Simmer for 1–1½ hours, or according to package instructions, until cooked and soft. Add extra water if necessary. Drain well and allow to cool.

2 Put the chickpeas, cherry tomatoes, celery, olives, and scallions in a serving bowl and mix well. Stir in the dressing, season with black pepper, garnish with mint leaves, and serve.

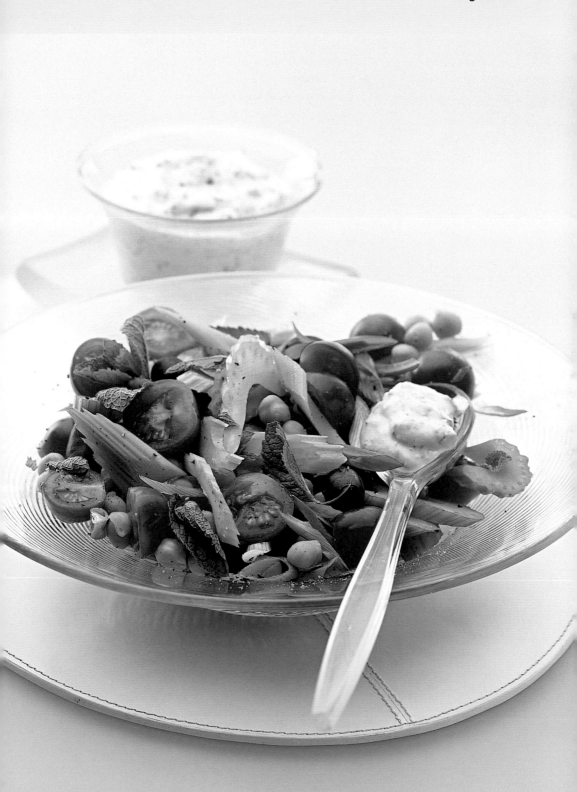

Nutritional values
Kcals 202 (846 Kj)
fat 13 g
saturated fat 3 g
sodium 280 mg
fiber 6 g

Preparation time
15 minutes
Cooking time
10 minutes
Serves
4

broiled eggplant with mint and yogurt dressing

2 tablespoons olive oil

2 eggplants, about 14½ ounces total weight, sliced thickly into rounds about ½ inch thick

freshly ground black pepper

DRESSING
1 small bunch of mint, chopped

2 garlic cloves, crushed

½ cup low-fat plain yogurt

⅓ cup reduced-fat hummus

1 To make the dressing, mix together the mint, crushed garlic, yogurt, and hummus.

2 Brush a baking sheet with a little of the olive oil and arrange the slices of eggplant on the sheet in a single layer—you may have to cook the eggplant in 2 batches if necessary. Brush the eggplant lightly with oil and place under a hot broiler. When the eggplant is soft and golden and beginning to char at the edges (after about 4–5 minutes), turn over the slices and cook the other side for another 3–4 minutes.

3 Lift the eggplants off the baking sheet and onto a warmed plate. Spoon the dressing over and serve with a chickpea salad (see page 96), if desired.

Nutritional values

Kcals 413 (1714 Kj)

fat 33 g

saturated fat 7 g

sodium 198 mg

fiber 7 g

Preparation time

10 minutes

Cooking time

25 minutes

Serves

4

NUTRITIONAL TIP

Packed with fresh vegetables, this dish is bursting with healthy nutrients. In addition, the yogurt in the dressing supplies calcium.

roasted vegetables with creamy arugula pesto sauce

2 red bell peppers, cored, seeded, and cut into bite-size pieces

1 yellow bell pepper, cored, seeded, and cut into bite-size pieces

1 large eggplant, cut into bite-size pieces

2 small red onions, quartered

2 large zucchini, sliced into bite-size pieces

1 head of garlic

4 tablespoons olive oil

7 ounces cherry tomatoes

freshly ground black pepper

whole wheat bread, to serve

PESTO DRESSING
1 cup arugula, chopped

1 garlic clove, peeled

1 cup freshly grated Parmesan cheese

6 tablespoons olive oil

⅓ cup low-fat plain bio yogurt

1 Place all the vegetables, except the tomatoes, in a large roasting pan. Separate the garlic cloves but don't peel them, then sprinkle them over the vegetables. Drizzle over the oil and mix well. Season with black pepper and place in a preheated oven, 425° F. After 20 minutes add the tomatoes and cook for an additional 5 minutes.

2 To make the pesto dressing, place the arugula, garlic, Parmesan, and olive oil in a food processor or blender and blend until smooth. Stir the pesto into the yogurt.

3 Transfer the roasted vegetables to a serving dish and serve with the pesto dressing and crusty whole wheat bread.

Nutritional values

Kcals 500 (2117 Kj)

fat 11 g

saturated fat 3 g

sodium 64 mg

fiber 17 g

Preparation time

10 minutes, plus

soaking

Cooking time

1 hour 35 minutes–2

hours 5 minutes

Serves

4

NUTRITIONAL TIP

Potassium is an important nutrient for everyone, particularly those with high blood pressure. All fruits and vegetables contain the mineral and this vegetable pilaf contains some of the best sources of all, for example, raisins, dried apricots, and tomatoes.

moroccan vegetable pilaf

4 ounces dried chickpeas, soaked overnight in cold water

1 tablespoon unsalted butter

1 cup long-grain rice

1 cardamom pod, crushed

1 cinnamon stick

3 cups low-sodium Vegetable stock (see page 102)

¼ cup raisins

1 tablespoon olive oil

1 red onion, sliced thinly

2 garlic cloves, crushed

½ teaspoon ground cumin

½–1 tablespoon harissa

¾ cup dried apricots, chopped roughly

2 large carrots, sliced thickly

1 red bell pepper, cored, seeded, and chopped roughly

7½ ounces cherry tomatoes

grated zest of 1 large orange

1 tablespoon slivered almonds

2 tablespoons roughly chopped fresh cilantro

freshly ground black pepper

1 Drain the chickpeas, rinse well and drain again. Put them into a large saucepan, cover with plenty of cold water and bring to the boil. Simmer for 1–1½ hours, or according to package instructions, until cooked and soft. Add extra water if necessary. Drain well and allow to cool.

2 Melt the butter in a large saucepan. Add the rice, cardamom, and cinnamon, and cook, stirring, for 1 minute. Stir in half the stock, ¼ cup of water, and the raisins. Bring to a boil, reduce the heat, and simmer for 20 minutes, then drain.

3 While the rice is cooking prepare the vegetables. Heat the oil in a large saucepan, add the red onion and cook for 5 minutes or until beginning to soften. Add the garlic, cumin, and harissa and cook for an additional 1 minute.

4 Add the apricots, carrots, and bell pepper to the pan and stir. Pour over the remaining stock and bring to a boil. Add black pepper to taste, cover, and simmer for 15 minutes.

5 Add the chickpeas and cherry tomatoes and cook for an additional 10 minutes or until the vegetables are just tender.

6 Stir the grated orange zest into the rice. Transfer the rice to a serving bowl and spoon over the vegetables. Lightly toast the almonds and sprinkle over, together with the cilantro, to serve.

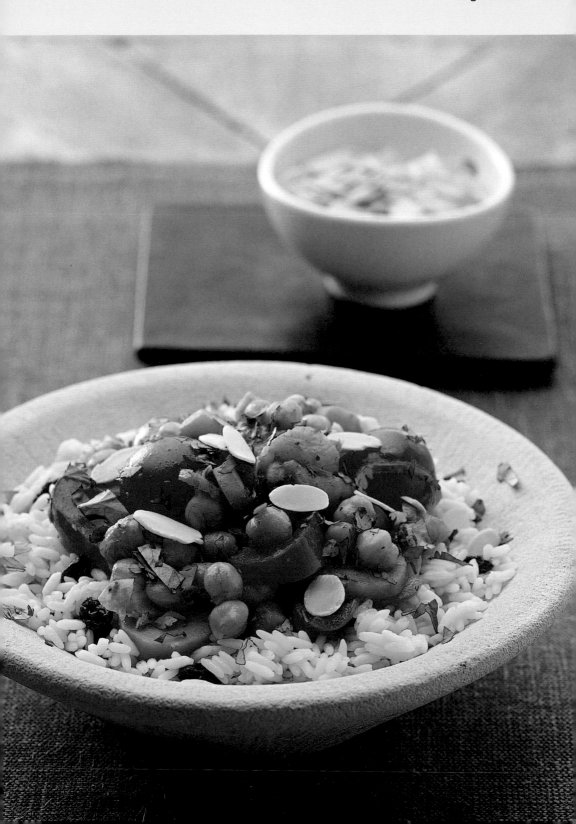

Nutritional values
Kcals 356 (1506 Kj)
fat 7 g
saturated fat 4 g
sodium 68 mg
fiber 5 g

Preparation time
10 minutes, plus
making the stock
Cooking time
35–40 minutes
Serves
4

leek and tomato risotto

2 tablespoons unsalted butter

13 ounces leeks, trimmed and sliced thinly

1½ cups Arborio rice

½ teaspoon paprika

½ teaspoon cayenne pepper

13-ounce can chopped tomatoes

freshly ground black pepper

shredded basil leaves

VEGETABLE STOCK
1 tablespoon olive oil

2 onions, chopped roughly

2 carrots, chopped roughly

1 pound mixed vegetables, such as parsnips, leeks, zucchini, mushrooms, and tomatoes

1 bouquet garni

1 teaspoon black peppercorns

1 First make the stock. Heat the oil in a large heavy saucepan and gently fry all the vegetables for 5 minutes. Add 6 cups cold water and bring slowly to a boil. Reduce the heat and simmer gently for 40 minutes, skimming occasionally. Skim the stock and allow to cool, then chill. Remove any fat from the surface before using.

2 Melt the butter in a large deep skillet. Add the leeks and cook for 3–4 minutes. Add the rice and spices and cook, stirring, for 1–2 minutes.

3 Heat the stock, then strain, and ladle out 5 cups. Add the tomatoes and hot stock to the rice and bring to a boil. Reduce the heat and simmer, stirring frequently, for 30 minutes. Add black pepper to taste, sprinkle over the shredded basil leaves and serve.

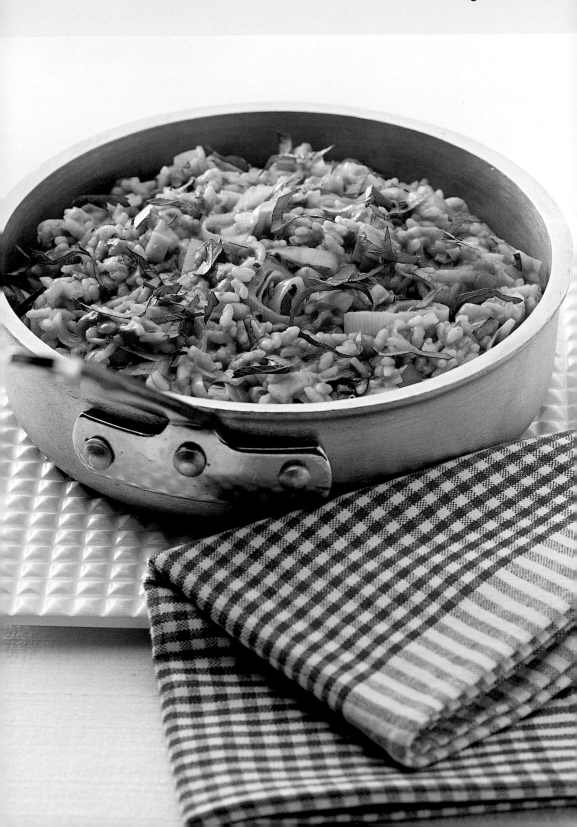

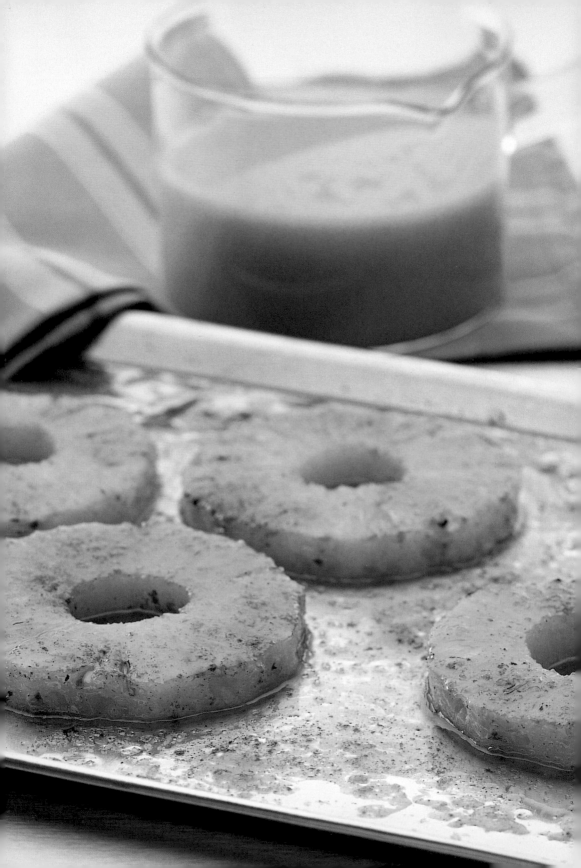

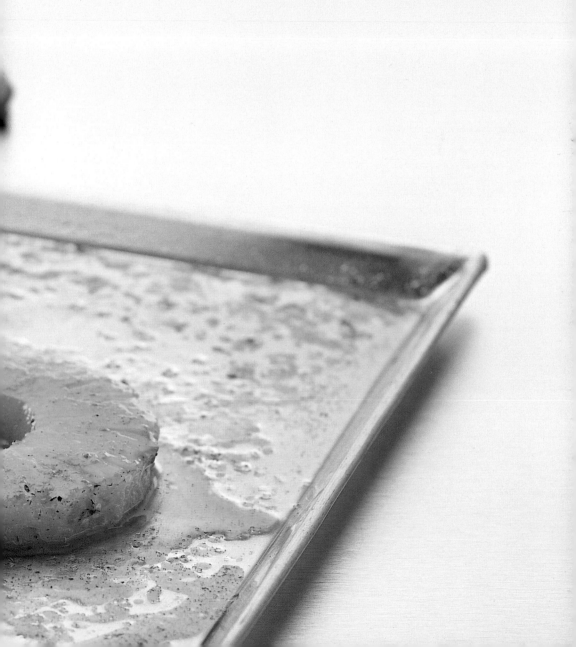

desserts

Nutritional values

Kcals 137 (583 Kj)

fat 0 g

saturated fat 0 g

sodium 23 mg

fiber 2 g

Preparation time

10 minutes, plus

standing and chilling

Cooking time

5 minutes

Serves

6

strawberry delights

1½ cups strawberries, hulled

½ cup caster sugar

2 cups white grape juice

3 envelopes gelatin, each
¼ ounce (or 6 leaves)

5 tablespoons cassis (optional)

1 Roughly chop three quarters of the strawberries and place in a food processor or blender with 1¼ cups boiling water and the sugar, and blend until smooth. Place the mixture in a strainer set over a bowl and stir to allow the liquid to drip through.

2 Pour ¾ cup of the grape juice into a small heatproof bowl, sprinkle over the gelatin and allow to stand for 10 minutes. Place the bowl over a saucepan of simmering water and stir until the gelatin has dissolved. Leave to cool then stir in the cassis, if using, strawberry liquid, and the remaining grape juice.

3 Arrange the remaining strawberries in 6 large wine glasses, pour over the liquid, and chill until set.

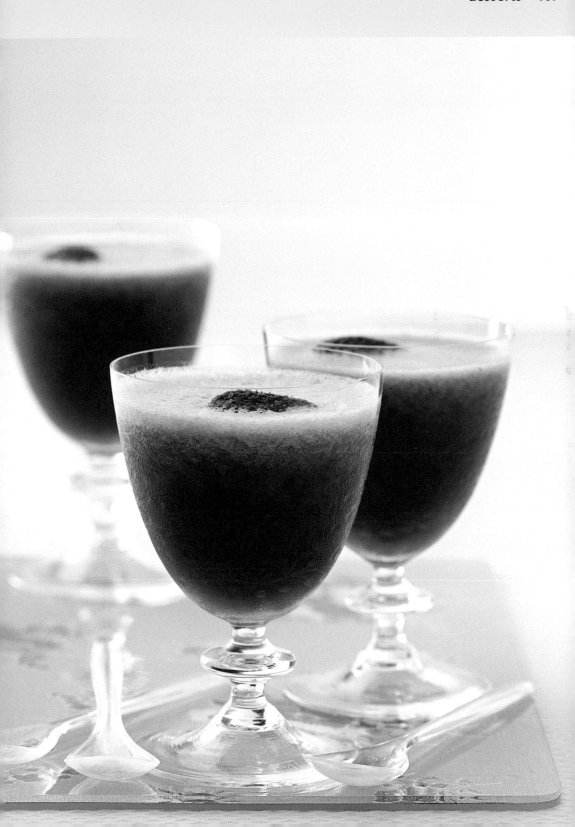

Nutritional values

Kcals 213 (911 Kj)

fat 0.5 g

saturated fat 0 g

sodium 30 mg

fiber 4.5 g

Preparation time

15 minutes, plus

cooling and chilling

Cooking time

10 minutes

Serves

4

✚ NUTRITIONAL TIP

Fruit salad is always a good choice when it comes to adopting a healthy eating plan. The lemongrass and ginger give this fruit salad a bit of a kick.

tropical fruit salad with ginger and lemongrass syrup

$\frac{1}{3}$ **cup superfine sugar**

1 lemongrass stalk, outer leaves removed, cut into 3 pieces, and each crushed with a rolling pin

1 piece of preserved ginger, chopped finely

1 galia or ogen melon, halved, seeded, and cubed

$\frac{1}{2}$ **ripe pineapple, peeled and cubed**

2 ripe mangoes, peeled and sliced

4 ripe kiwi fruit, peeled and sliced

cape gooseberries, to decorate (optional)

1 Place the sugar, lemongrass, and $\frac{2}{3}$ cup water in a small heavy saucepan and heat gently until the sugar dissolves. Bring to a boil and simmer for 5 minutes. Allow the syrup to cool for 10 minutes then remove and discard the lemongrass and stir in the chopped ginger.

2 Place the prepared fruit in a serving bowl, pour over the syrup, and chill.

3 To serve, peel back the papery husks of the cape gooseberries to form "flowers." Sprinkle over the top of the fruit salad to decorate.

Nutritional values

Kcals 209 (888 Kj)

fat 0 g

saturated fat 0 g

sodium 5 mg

fiber 3 g

Preparation time

10 minutes, plus chilling

Cooking time

20 minutes

Serves

4

pears poached with star anise

4 firm ripe pears

grated zest and juice of 1 large lemon

⅔ cup sugar

2 star anise

1 Peel the pears but leave the stalks intact. Place the lemon juice and zest, sugar, 2½ cups water, and star anise in a saucepan. Bring to a boil and stir gently until the sugar dissolves.

2 Reduce the heat to a gentle simmer. Add the pears, cover, and simmer for 15 minutes or until the pears are tender.

3 Remove the pears from the pan. Turn the heat up high and boil the remaining liquid until it starts to become thick and syrupy. Pour the hot syrup over the pears, allow to cool, then refrigerate for at least 1 hour before serving.

Nutritional values

Kcals 340 (1428 Kj)

fat 14 g

saturated fat 7 g

sodium 165 mg

fiber 3 g

Preparation time

15 minutes,

plus cooling

Cooking time

15 minutes

Serves

4

NUTRITIONAL TIP

Bananas are a very rich source of potassium, the mineral that helps regulate blood pressure. Here they are combined with sesame seeds, which lower the risk of heart disease and stroke and help reduce high blood pressure.

banana and cardamom phyllo parcels

3 tablespoons raw brown sugar

3 large bananas, sliced

¼ cup unsalted butter

½ teaspoon ground cardamom

4 sheets phyllo pastry, 16 x 11 inches

1 tablespoon sesame seeds

Low-fat plain yogurt, to serve

1 Sprinkle the sugar over the bananas. Melt half the butter in a saucepan, add the sugary bananas and cook over a low heat for 10 minutes. Remove from the heat, stir in the ground cardamom, and allow to cool.

2 Melt the remaining butter. Lay one sheet of phyllo on a clean countertop, brush lightly with a little melted butter, then fold into three lengthwise. Spoon a quarter of the banana mixture onto the pastry about 1½ inches from the end. Fold the left corner of the phyllo diagonally to the right side of the dough to cover the filling. Continue folding in the same way until you reach the end of the sheet. Repeat the process with the remaining sheets of phyllo. Place the turnovers on a lightly greased baking sheet, brush with a little more melted butter, and sprinkle over the sesame seeds.

3 Bake the turnovers in a preheated oven, 400° F., for 15 minutes or until golden. Serve with a spoonful of yogurt.

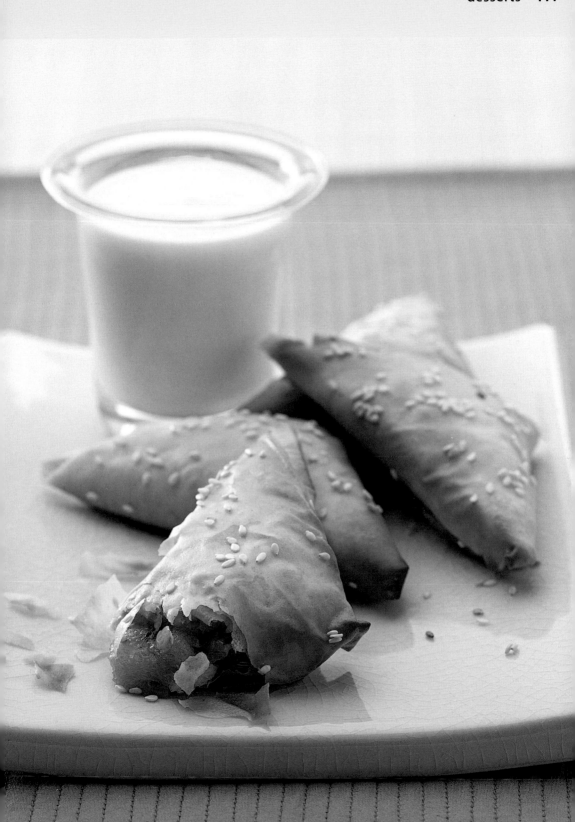

Nutritional values
Kcals 539 (2260 Kj)
fat 27 g
saturated fat 17 g
sodium 47 mg
fiber 7 g

Preparation time
10 minutes
Cooking time
45 minutes
Serves
4–6

rhubarb and strawberry crumble

1 pound 6 ounces rhubarb, trimmed and cut into 1-inch lengths

⅓ cup elderflower cordial

2 cups fresh or frozen strawberries, thawed if frozen

¼ cup superfine sugar

Low-fat plain yogurt or soya cream alternative to serve

CRUMBLE
1 cup all-purpose flour

½ cup rolled oats

½ cup unsalted butter, diced

¼ cup superfine sugar

1 To make the crumble topping, place the flour and oats in a bowl and blend in the butter until the mixture resembles bread crumbs. Stir in the sugar.

2 Place the rhubarb in a shallow ovenproof dish. Pour over the elderflower cordial, cover the dish with foil, and place in a preheated oven, 400° F., for 10 minutes, or until the rhubarb is just tender. Stir in the strawberries, together with a little sugar if necessary.

3 Place the crumble mixture on top of the fruit, pressing it down firmly to get a nice compact topping. Bake in the oven for 35 minutes, or until the crumble has turned golden brown. Serve hot with yogurt or soya cream.

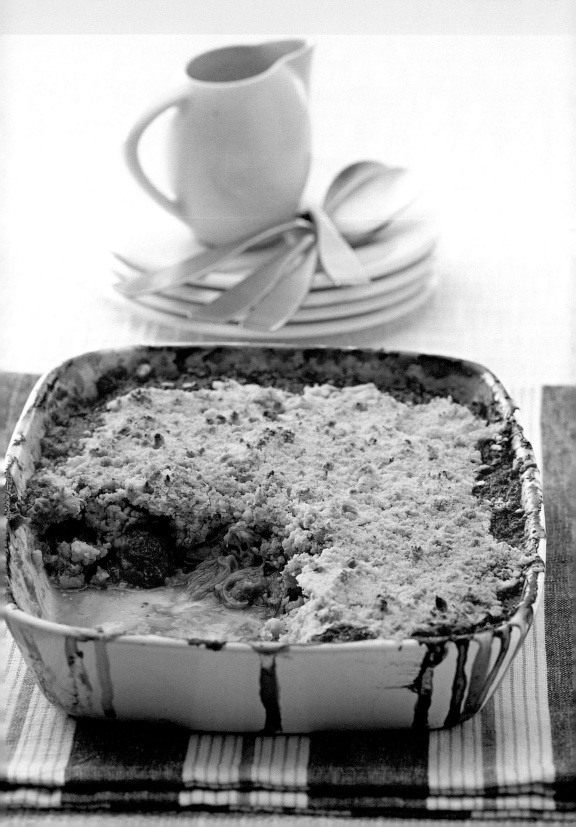

Nutritional values

Kcals 125 (532 Kj)

fat 3 g

saturated fat 2 g

sodium 13 mg

fiber 3 g

Preparation time

15 minutes

Cooking time

20 minutes

Serves

4

caramelized pineapple
with apricot coulis

8 fresh apricots, pitted

¾ cup orange juice

4 teaspoons raw brown sugar, plus extra to taste

1 teaspoon mixed spice

1 tablespoon unsalted butter, melted

4 thick slices of fresh pineapple, peeled and cored

mint sprigs and cape gooseberries, to decorate

1 Roughly chop the apricots and place in a saucepan with the orange juice. Cook over a low heat for 10–15 minutes or until quite soft. Transfer to a blender and blend until smooth, adding a little sugar to taste and a little more orange juice if necessary.

2 Combine the mixed spice and melted butter. Place the slices of pineapple on a baking sheet covered with foil. Brush the pineapple with the spiced melted butter, sprinkle over the sugar and cook under a preheated medium hot broiler for 2–3 minutes on each side.

3 Place the pineapple on plates, pour over a little of the apricot sauce, and serve warm, decorated with mint sprigs and a few cape gooseberries.

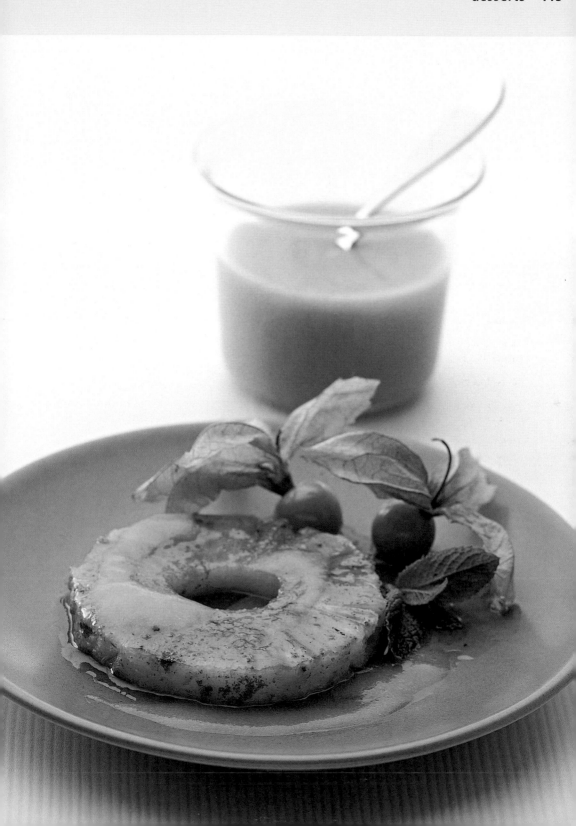

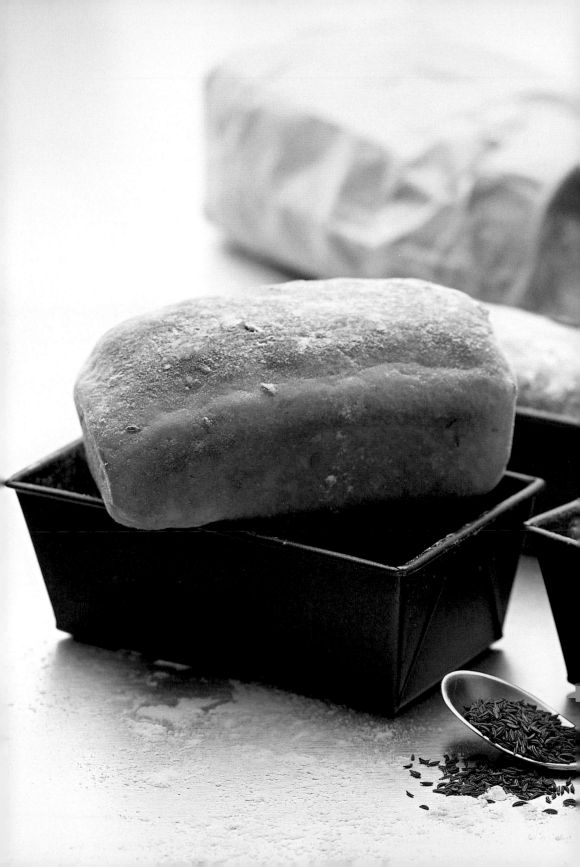

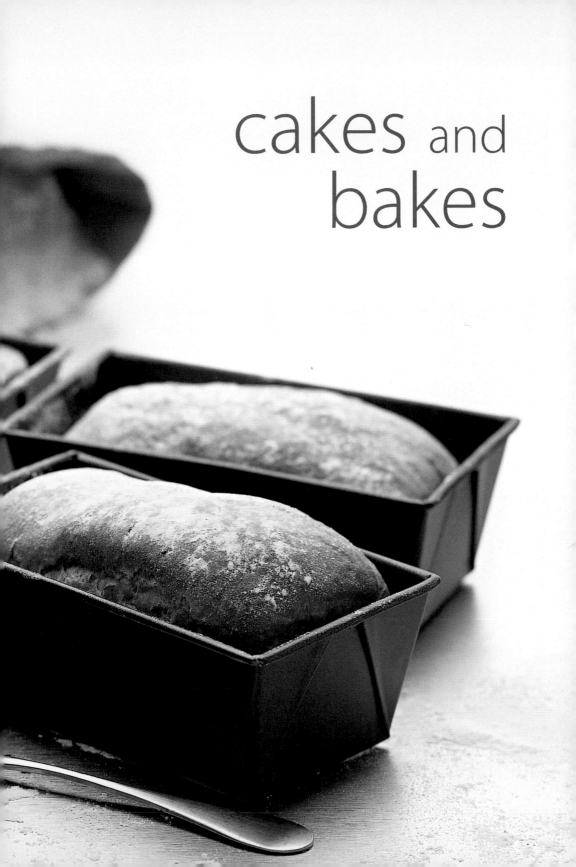

cakes and
bakes

Nutritional values

Kcals 269 (1126 Kj)

fat 16 g

saturated fat 1 g

sodium 60 mg

fiber 2 g

Preparation time

10 minutes

Cooking time

30–35 minutes

Serves

12

 NUTRITIONAL TIP

Like all dried fruit, dates are a good natural source of potassium, while the pecan nuts provide essential fatty acids. Both nutrients are known to be effective in regulating blood pressure.

sticky fruit and nut bars

¾ **cup roughly chopped pitted dates**

¼ **cup raw brown sugar**

½ **cup all-purpose flour**

½ **cup rolled oats**

1 **teaspoon baking powder**

1 **teaspoon ground cinnamon**

1½ **cups roughly chopped pecan nuts**

2 **large eggs, beaten**

4 **tablespoons canola oil**

4 **tablespoons reduced-sugar rough-cut marmalade or apricot jelly**

1 Place all the dry ingredients in a large bowl and mix well. Stir in the beaten eggs and canola oil and mix well.

2 Pour the mixture into a 6-inch square pan lined with waxed paper. Level the top and bake in a preheated oven, 350° F., for 30–35 minutes, or until the top is firm. Allow to cool in the pan for 10 minutes, then turn onto a wire rack to cool.

3 Heat the marmalade or apricot jelly in a small saucepan and brush over the top of the cake. When cold cut into 12 bars. The bars can be stored in an airtight container for up to 5 days.

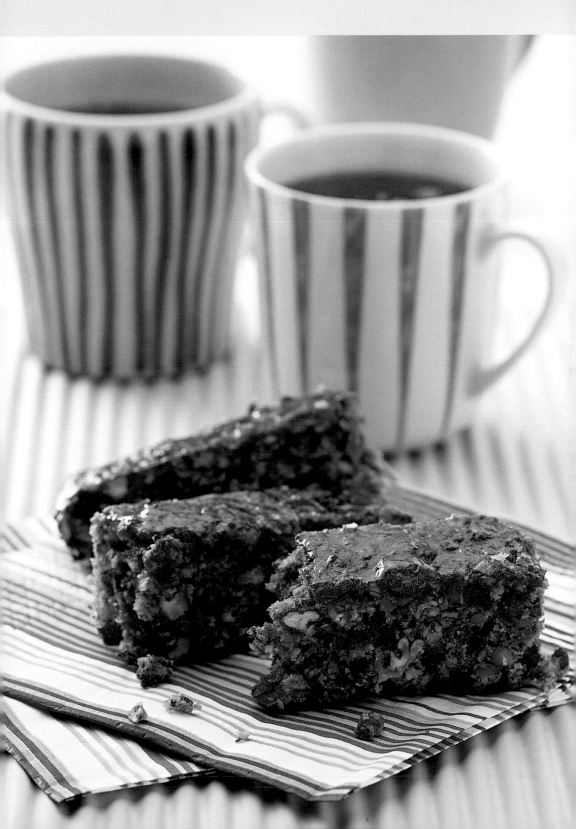

Nutritional values

Kcals 208 (886 Kj)

fat 1 g

saturated fat 0 g

sodium 115 mg

fiber 6 g

Preparation time

15 minutes,

plus standing

Cooking time

1 hour

Makes

10 slices

NUTRITIONAL TIP

Dried fruits are an excellent source of potassium, which helps remove excess sodium from the body and reduce high blood pressure.

ginger teabread

⅔ **cup ready-to-eat dried apricots, chopped roughly**

⅔ **cup ready-to-eat dried prunes, chopped roughly**

¾ **cup roughly chopped dried figs**

1¼ **cups hot Earl Grey tea**

1 **tablespoon preserved ginger**

1 **teaspoon ground ginger**

2 **cups all-purpose flour**

2 **teaspoons baking powder**

½ **cup granulated dark brown sugar**

1 **egg, beaten**

2 **tablespoons cold water**

1 Place the dried fruit in a large heatproof bowl. Pour over the tea and allow to stand for at least 2 hours, or preferably overnight, stirring occasionally.

2 Place the fruit and all the remaining ingredients in a large bowl and mix together thoroughly. Turn the mixture into a lightly greased and base-lined 2-pound loaf pan. Level the surface and brush lightly with 2 tablespoons cold water.

3 Cook in a preheated oven, 350° F., for 1 hour, or until the cake feels springy in the center. If necessary cover with foil after 30 minutes to prevent the top from burning.

4 Allow the cake to cool in the pan for 10–15 minutes. Loosen the edges with a knife then turn out onto a wire rack to cool. The cake can be stored in an airtight container for up to a week.

Nutritional values

Kcals 353 (1476 Kj)

fat 21 g

saturated fat 8 g

sodium 128 mg

fiber 3 g

Preparation time

15 minutes

Cooking time

45 minutes

Serves

10

 NUTRITIONAL TIP

Ensuring you have a good intake of potassium and essential fatty acids is a good step toward controlling your blood pressure. The ingredients in this teabread are a good source of both of them.

banana and pecan teabread

1⅓ **cups whole wheat flour**

½ **cup all-purpose flour**

½ **cup unsalted butter or polyunsaturated margarine**

½ **cup dark brown sugar**

2 **teaspoons baking powder**

¼ **teaspoon ground cinnamon**

2 **large eggs, beaten**

3 **ripe bananas, about 12 ounces, peeled and mashed**

1 **cup roughly chopped pecan nuts**

1 Place all the ingredients except the banana and pecans in a large bowl and, using an electric hand beater, beat the mixture until evenly mixed. Stir in the banana and pecans, taking care not to overmix.

2 Spoon the mixture into a lightly greased and base-lined 2-pound loaf pan. Bake in a preheated oven, 350° F., for 45 minutes, or until the cake feels springy in the center. You may need to cover the cake with foil halfway through cooking to prevent it burning. Allow the cake to cool in the pan for 5 minutes then carefully turn out onto a wire rack. The teabread can be stored in an airtight container for up to 5 days.

Nutritional values

Kcals 313 (1314 Kj)

fat 17 g

saturated fat 7 g

sodium 111 mg

fiber 2 g

Preparation time

15 minutes

Cooking time

30 minutes

Makes

12–14 slices

NUTRITIONAL TIP

Walnuts are beneficial to overall health, and particularly the heart, being rich in both Omega-3 and Omega-6 essential fatty acids.

apple and walnut streusel cake

2 cups self-rising flour

$^1/_2$ cup unsalted butter, softened

$^3/_4$ cup golden raisins

$^1/_2$ cup granulated light brown sugar

1 cup roughly chopped walnuts

2 eggs

2 tablespoons semi-skimmed milk

TOPPING
2 dessert apples, cored and sliced

$^1/_4$ cup self-rising flour, sifted

1 tablespoon unsalted butter, at room temperature

2 tablespoons raw brown sugar

$^1/_2$ teaspoon ground cinnamon

2 teaspoons cold water

1 Place all the cake ingredients in a bowl and beat together until smooth. Spoon into an 7 x 11-inch shallow pan lined with parchment paper, and spread out.

2 To make the topping, arrange the apple slices on top of the cake mixture. Place the flour in a bowl and blend in the butter until the mixture resembles fine bread crumbs. Add the sugar and cinnamon. Stir in 2 teaspoons cold water and mix well. Spread over the slices of apple.

3 Bake in the center of a preheated oven, 350° F., for 30 minutes, or until the cake feels set when lightly pressed in the center.

4 Remove from the oven and allow to cool in the pan for 5–10 minutes, then transfer to a wire rack and allow to cool completely. The cake can be stored in an airtight container for up to 5 days.

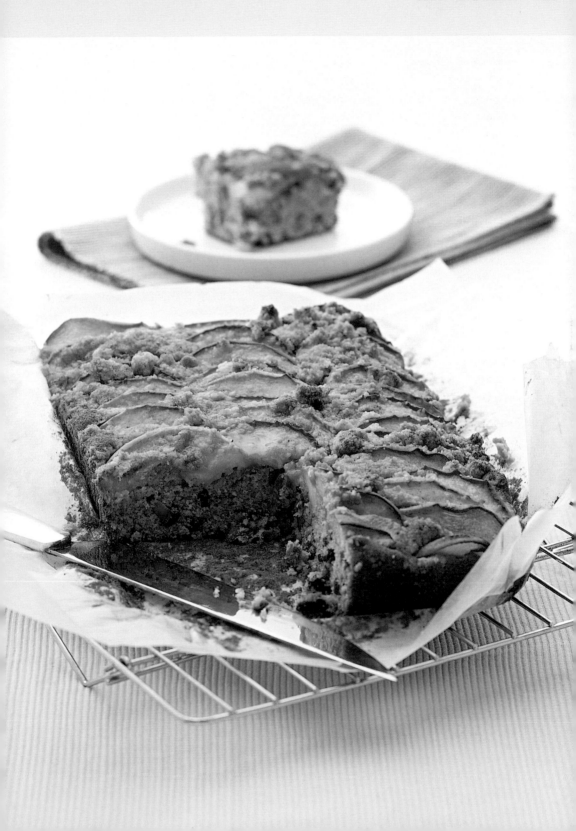

Nutritional values
Kcals 476 (2011 Kj)
fat 24 g
saturated fat 6 g
sodium 258 mg
fiber 5 g

Preparation time
15 minutes
Cooking time
1¼–1½ hours
Serves
8–10

spiced zucchini teabread

1¾ cups whole wheat self-rising flour

1 tablespoon ground mixed spice

1 teaspoon baking soda

1¼ cups granulated dark brown sugar

⅔ cup sunflower oil

grated zest and juice of 1 large orange

2 eggs, beaten

2 zucchini, about 8 ounces, grated coarsely

½ cup roughly chopped walnuts

¾ cup golden raisins

⅔ cup shredded coconut

1 tablespoon lemon juice

1 Mix together the flour, ground mixed spice, and baking soda. In another bowl beat 1 cup of the sugar with the sunflower oil and the orange zest until smooth. Gradually beat in the eggs until the mixture is light and creamy. Beat in the flour mixture, then stir in the zucchini, walnuts, golden raisins, and coconut.

2 Spoon the mixture into a lightly greased and base-lined 2-pound loaf pan. Bake in the center of a preheated oven, 325° F., for 1¼–1½ hours or until cooked. Check the cake is cooked by inserting a thin metal skewer into the middle of it. When the cake is cooked the skewer will come out clean.

3 To make the syrup, place the orange juice with the remaining sugar and the lemon juice in a small saucepan and heat until the sugar dissolves. Boil for 1 minute then remove from the heat.

4 Using a toothpick, prick the cake in several places then drizzle over the syrup. When cool, the cake can be stored in an airtight container for up to 5 days.

Nutritional values
Kcals 140 (598 Kj)
fat 0.6 g
saturated fat 0.1 g
sodium 73 mg
fiber 2 g

Preparation time
30 minutes, plus rising
Cooking time
30–35 minutes
Makes
6 x 1-pound loaves
or 3 x 2-pound loaves

low-sodium bread

5 cups bread flour

1 envelope easy-blend yeast

1 tablespoon superfine sugar

1 tablespoon caraway seeds

½ teaspoon salt

1¼ cups buttermilk

1 Place half of the flour, the yeast, sugar, caraway seeds, and salt in a large bowl. Place the buttermilk and 2 tablespoons water in a saucepan and heat until tepid; be careful not to overheat, as you will kill the yeast when you add it to the flour.

2 Gradually beat the buttermilk mixture into the flour with a wooden spoon until it becomes a thick batter. Beat in the remaining flour to make a thick dough.

3 Tip out onto a lightly floured surface and knead for 10 minutes until smooth.

4 Grease either 6 x 1-pound loaf pans or 3 x 2-pound loaf pans. Divide the mixture into the prepared pans, cover with a clean dish towel and leave in a warm place for about 1 hour or until the mixture has doubled in size.

5 Uncover and transfer to a preheated oven, 375° F., and bake for 30–35 minutes or until each loaf sounds hollow when tapped. Remove the loaves from the pans and cool on a wire rack.

index

acknowledgments

Executive Editor: Nicky Hill
Editor: Jessica Cowie
Executive Art Editor: Rozelle Bentheim
Designer: Beverly Price, one2six creative
Home Ecomony: Bethany Heald/David Morgan
Production Controller: Nigel Reed

picture credits

Special Photography: © Octopus Publishing Group/William Lingwood

Getty Images 11 top, 20 left, 29 top right, 31 right, 34
Octopus Publishing Group Limited 11 bottom /Stephen Conroy 34 /
Marcus Harpur 29 bottom right /Peter Myers 33 right /William Reavell
12 right, 25 bottom right, 32 top, 32 bottom /Gareth Sambidge 26 left